# the natural
# PREGNANCY BOOK

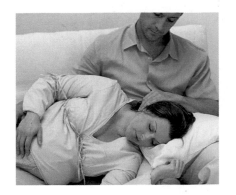

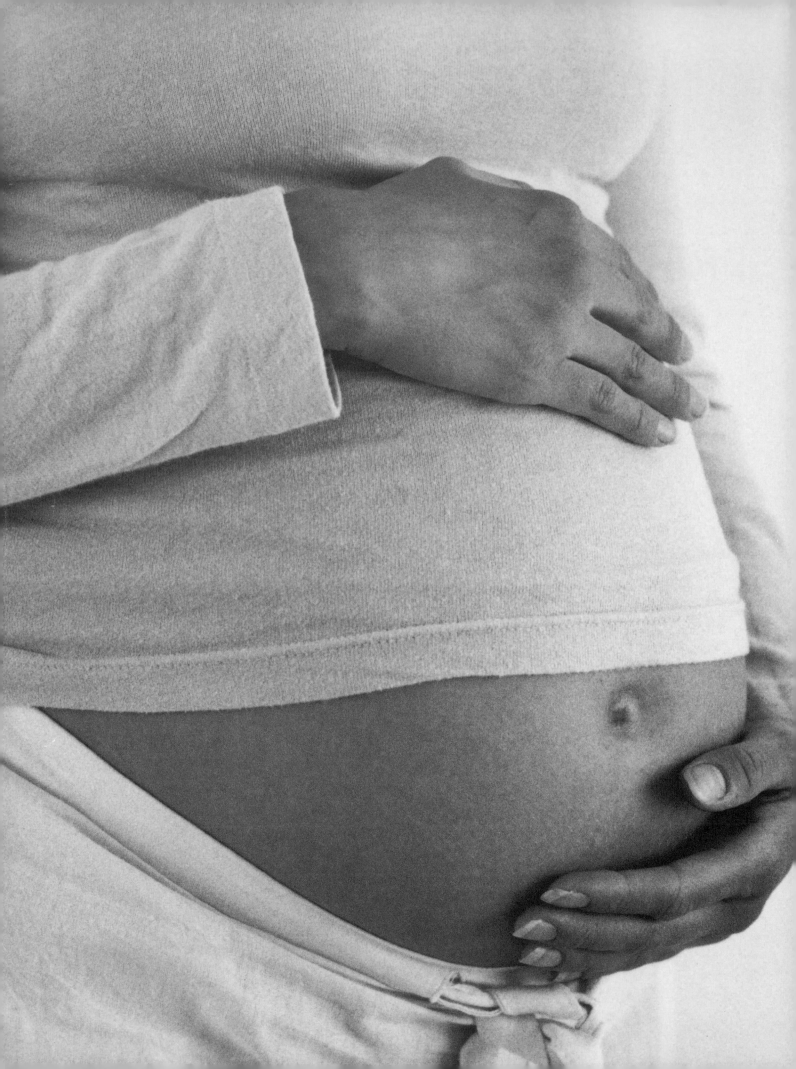

# the natural
# PREGNANCY BOOK

How to have a happy, healthy pregnancy and birth – all the
medical facts explained, plus sensible eating and exercise plans and
gentle supportive therapies, from homeopathy to meditation

**Anne Charlish**
and Kim Davies

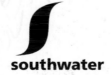

**southwater**

This edition is published by Southwater
an imprint of Anness Publishing Ltd
Blaby Road, Wigston
Leicestershire LE18 4SE
info@anness.com

www.southwaterbooks.com;
www.annesspublishing.com

Anness Publishing has a new picture agency outlet
for images for publishing, promotions or advertising.
Please visit our website www.practicalpictures.com
for more information.

Publisher **Joanna Lorenz**
Editorial Director **Helen Sudell**
Project Editor **Ann Kay**
Copy Editor **Kim Davies**
Designer **Lisa Tai**
Special Photography **Alistair Hughes**
Illustrations **Sam Elmhurst**
Production Controller **Wendy Lawson**

© Anness Publishing Ltd 2012

A CIP catalogue record for this book is available from
the British Library.

**PUBLISHER'S NOTE**
The information in this book and the opinions of the
authors should not be regarded as a substitute for
attention from a qualified health professional. If you
are suffering from any medical complaint, or are
worried about any aspect of your health, you must
get a medical opinion.

Always seek advice before starting any exercise
programme, whether you are pregnant or not, but
especially during pregnancy. The publishers can take
no responsibility for any kind of injury or illness
resulting from the advice given or the exercises and
routines demonstrated in this book.

At the time of writing, the authors had made every
effort, as far as they were able, to ensure that the
information in this book was accurate, up to date and
in accordance with current practices and guidelines.

# contents

Introduction    6

**CHAPTER 1**

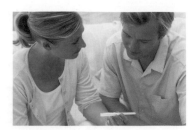

## The First Trimester

The First Trimester    8
Confirming pregnancy    10
Early development    12
Development from six weeks    14
How your body is changing    16
Emotional changes    18
Pregnancy and eating    20
Avoiding toxic substances    24
Good ways to exercise    26
Keeping your joints mobile    28
Yoga for the first trimester    30
Creating a balanced life    32
Routine antenatal care    34
Tests and specialist care    36
Possible problems    38
Checklist of common problems    40
Common Qs and As    42

**CHAPTER 2**

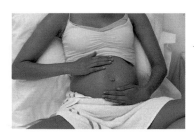

## The Second Trimester

The Second Trimester    44
Growth from twelve weeks    46
How your body is changing    50
Emotional changes    52
Aromatherapy for pregnancy    54
Massage relief    56
How to massage yourself    58
Treating ailments at home    60
Yoga for the second trimester    62
Pregnancy and your sex life    64
Routine antenatal care    66
Tests and procedures    68
Amniocentesis in perspective    70
When something is wrong    72
Checklist of common problems    74
Common Qs and As    76

CHAPTER

3

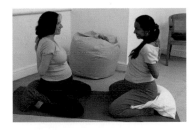

## The Third Trimester 78
How your baby is developing 80
How your body is changing 82
Emotional changes 84
Feel-good treats and therapies 86
Perineal and breast massage 88
Yoga for the third trimester 90
Hip-openers in water 92
Antenatal care 94
Antenatal classes 96
Checklist of common problems 98
Common Qs and As 100

CHAPTER

4

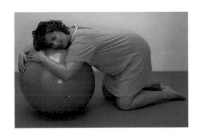

## Countdown to Birth 102
Your birth plan 104
Where to have your baby 106
Giving birth in water 108
Preparing for the birth 110
What your baby will need 112
Before the birth 114
Going into labour 116
Pain relief and monitoring 118
The first stage of labour 120
The second and third stages 122
Medical interventions 124
Checklist of common problems 126
Common Qs and As 128

CHAPTER

5

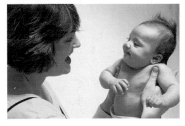

## You and Your New Baby 130
Meeting your new baby 132
Feeding your baby 134
Changing and bathing 138
Coping with the early days 140
Checklist of common problems 142
Common Qs and As 144

CHAPTER

6

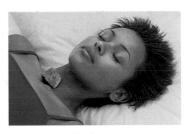

## Natural Therapies 146
Herbalism and Homeopathy 148
Aromatherapy and Massage 149
Acupuncture, Shiatsu and Reflexology 150
Meditation (including hypnotherapy), Reiki,
    Colour Therapy and Crystal Healing 151
Feng shui and T'ai chi 152
Yoga and Pilates 153
Alexander Technique, Osteopathy
    and Chiropractic 154
Which therapy? 155

Glossary 156
Useful addresses and websites 158
Index 159
Acknowledgements 160

# Introduction

" This book will give you all you need to ensure that your pregnancy is as wonderful, natural and personal as it can be. "

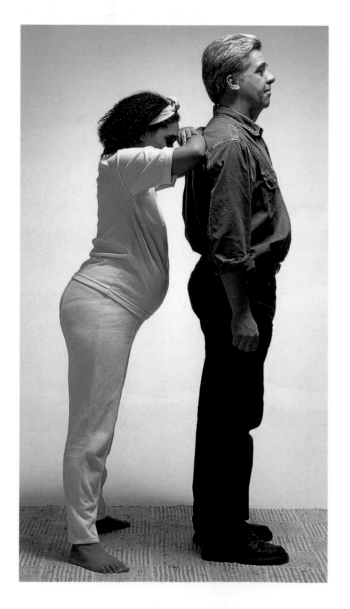

There are two main aspects to pregnancy. On the one hand, there are the medical matters. Scientific know-how has made pregnancy and birth extremely safe, and a mother-to-be can very well entrust herself to the care of doctors. On the other hand, pregnancy is a major life experience where your personality, your ideas about parenting and the feelings you have about your own body are all highly significant.

This book aims to give you the best of both the medical and the natural, holistic approaches. It tells you everything you need to know about the common obstetric procedures, but also emphasizes the importance of nutrition, exercise and a host of supportive complementary therapies – from yoga and homeopathy to meditation and herbalism.

This book will show you all kinds of ways in which you can help to give yourself the best chance of a happy pregnancy, a successful birth and a healthy baby. These pages guide you through every step of this extraordinary life event, from confirming the conception through each of the three main trimesters

*Partners, close friends and relatives can play a vital supportive role. Here, a woman practises using her partner for support during labour.*

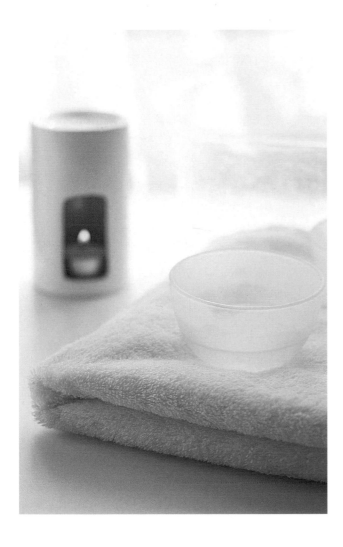

*All kinds of holistic therapies can assist women through every stage of pregnancy and childbirth – even if it is simply burning aromatic oils to create a calm and serene atmosphere.*

of pregnancy and on to giving birth and how to care for your new baby in his or her first few weeks of life. It explains clearly exactly what is happening to your body at each stage and gives you the answers to the most commonly asked questions. It also details the different choices that are available – the benefits that they can bring and the potential risks. For example, natural childbirth options are explained, but the book also advises on the drugs that are available if you decide you need them.

In the end you will decide for yourself just how you deal with the ups-and-downs, the joys and pains of pregnancy and childbirth. Rather than tell you what you must do, this book will give you all you need to make informed choices and to ensure that your pregnancy is every bit as wonderful, natural and personal as it can be.

## TAKE CARE

This book has been written with the aim of offering a wide range of help and advice to pregnant women. However, it is important to remember that no book can be a substitute for getting advice about your own medical circumstances. For this reason, all the suggestions in this book should be used under the guidance of your doctor and complementary practitioner.

If you are at all worried by any symptom during your pregnancy, or if you are unsure of whether or not a natural therapy is safe, do not hesitate to consult your family doctor.

You should call the emergency services and then sit down and wait for the ambulance to arrive if you notice any of the following:

- Vaginal bleeding, unless it is merely spotting.
- Severe abdominal pain, especially if you are also bleeding vaginally.
- Continuous and severe headache, with or without blurred vision and with or without swelling of the hands and ankles.
- Excessive vomiting in which you cannot keep down any food or liquid, even water.
- Breaking of the waters.
- After week 22 of your pregnancy, no fetal movements for longer than 12 hours.

Telephone your family doctor without delay if you notice any of these symptoms:

- A temperature of 38.5°C (101°F) or more.
- Sudden swelling of the hands and ankles. If you also have blurred vision and/or severe headache as well as the swelling, you should call an ambulance (see above).
- Urinating not only frequently (which is normal during pregnancy) but with pain as well when you pass water, as this usually signifies some kind of infection.

# CHAPTER ONE
# The first trimester

*" Having a baby is one of the most exciting experiences that you will ever have. "*

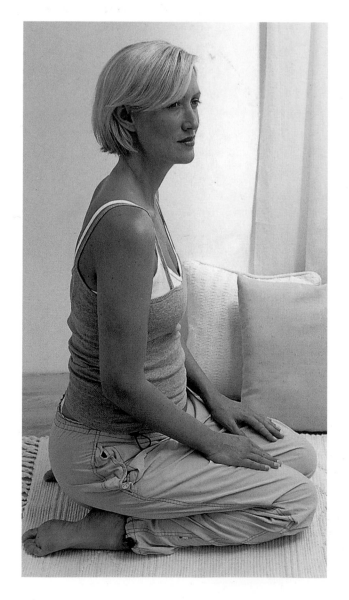

The first term of pregnancy, known as the first trimester, is roughly the first three months. This is an immensely thrilling time for a couple who have decided they want to start a family.

You and your partner will undoubtedly have many questions. Hopefully, this book will answer the majority of them but you should not hesitate to see your family doctor if you have any persistent worries. You will gain understanding, too, from your own experience. As every day passes, you will learn more about your body, your feelings about the pregnancy and the new life that you will soon be introducing into the world.

Pregnant women often experience minor physical disorders such as nausea and backache. There are often simple measures that you can take to relieve any discomfort that you may have, leaving you free to enjoy your pregnancy. In particular, complementary therapies can help to alleviate many

*The first 12 or 13 weeks of pregnancy is known as the first trimester. Many women have hardly any visible signs at all, while others do start to 'show'.*

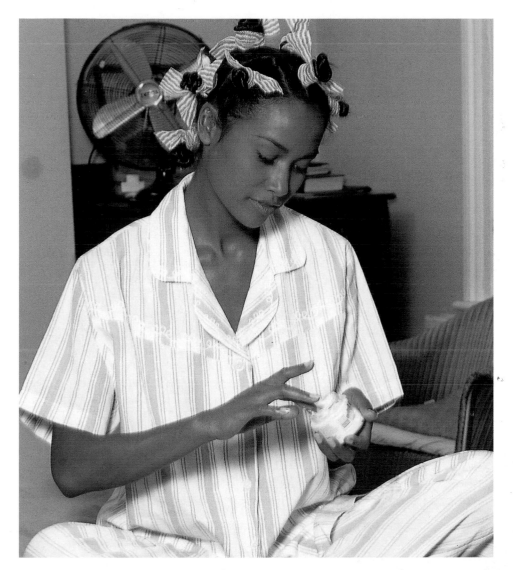

*Don't stint on pampering yourself whenever you can, and get plenty of rest and relaxation.*

*What you eat and drink remains as important as ever in these early formative weeks. Make sure you get your five portions of fruit and vegetables each day. Freshly squeezed fruit and vegetable juices are an especially enjoyable way to include these in your daily diet.*

pregnancy-related complaints and also enhance your well-being. The information in Chapter Six will help you to choose the therapy that is most suitable for you.

Having a baby is one of the most exciting experiences that you will ever have. These few weeks are precious, not least because you and your partner will see your baby's heart beating on ultrasound for the first time. This is living proof of the new life within you.

Don't forget that your body needs at least the first 12 weeks to adjust to this new state. As your hormonal balance shifts and you experience a whole new range of feelings, look after yourself as much as possible – put yourself and your baby first.

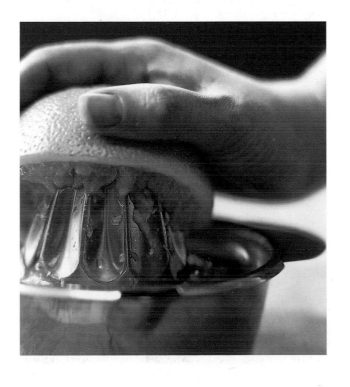

# Confirming pregnancy

Some women believe that they sensed the conception of their babies: they did not need to wait for a missed period or other symptoms to know that they were pregnant. This feeling could simply be intuition, or it is possible that these women are able to detect tiny changes inside the body that are associated with the first secretions of the pregnancy hormones. However, most women cannot be sure that they are pregnant until they have had it confirmed by a pregnancy test.

## EARLY SIGNS AND SYMPTOMS

The first definite sign of pregnancy is a missed period, known medically as amenorrhoea. Pregnancy is the most likely reason for a missed period, but it is not the only one – stress is another possible explanation. It is therefore best not to assume that you are pregnant just because you have missed your period. The following signs are other early indicators of pregnancy, some of which may occur before you miss a period. However, many women do not notice them until later in the pregnancy:

- Increased tiredness.
- Feeling nauseous, particularly in the mornings.
- Urinating more frequently than usual.
- Tenderness in the breasts.
- Changes in taste, such as a sudden craving for a particular food or a metallic taste in the mouth.

## CONFIRMING A PREGNANCY

Most women do their first pregnancy test at home. Pregnancy-testing kits are available from any pharmacy, and they are very accurate. The tests work by measuring the amount of one of the pregnancy hormones, human chorionic gonadotrophin (HCG), in your urine. If enough HCG is present, it triggers a reaction in the test. This is

---

### WHEN YOUR BABY IS DUE

If you know the date of your last period, you can work out your estimated date of delivery using the chart below. The delivery date is normally 40 weeks from the date of your last period but it can be up to two weeks earlier or later. A delivery outside those dates would be considered premature or post-mature.

| MONTH | ESTIMATED DATE OF DELIVERY | | | | | | | | | | | | | | | | | | | | | | | | | | | | | | | MONTH |
|---|---|---|---|---|---|---|---|---|---|---|---|---|---|---|---|---|---|---|---|---|---|---|---|---|---|---|---|---|---|---|---|---|
| January | 1 | 2 | 3 | 4 | 5 | 6 | 7 | 8 | 9 | 10 | 11 | 12 | 13 | 14 | 15 | 16 | 17 | 18 | 19 | 20 | 21 | 22 | 23 | 24 | 25 | 26 | 27 | 28 | 29 | 30 | 31 | January |
| October | 8 | 9 | 10 | 11 | 12 | 13 | 14 | 15 | 16 | 17 | 18 | 19 | 20 | 21 | 22 | 23 | 24 | 25 | 26 | 27 | 28 | 29 | 30 | 31 | 1 | 2 | 3 | 4 | 5 | 6 | 7 | November |
| February | 1 | 2 | 3 | 4 | 5 | 6 | 7 | 8 | 9 | 10 | 11 | 12 | 13 | 14 | 15 | 16 | 17 | 18 | 19 | 20 | 21 | 22 | 23 | 24 | 25 | 26 | 27 | 28 | | | | February |
| November | 8 | 9 | 10 | 11 | 12 | 13 | 14 | 15 | 16 | 17 | 18 | 19 | 20 | 21 | 22 | 23 | 24 | 25 | 26 | 27 | 28 | 29 | 30 | 1 | 2 | 3 | 4 | 5 | | | | December |
| March | 1 | 2 | 3 | 4 | 5 | 6 | 7 | 8 | 9 | 10 | 11 | 12 | 13 | 14 | 15 | 16 | 17 | 18 | 19 | 20 | 21 | 22 | 23 | 24 | 25 | 26 | 27 | 28 | 29 | 30 | 31 | March |
| December | 6 | 7 | 8 | 9 | 10 | 11 | 12 | 13 | 14 | 15 | 16 | 17 | 18 | 19 | 20 | 21 | 22 | 23 | 24 | 25 | 26 | 27 | 28 | 29 | 30 | 31 | 1 | 2 | 3 | 4 | 5 | January |
| April | 1 | 2 | 3 | 4 | 5 | 6 | 7 | 8 | 9 | 10 | 11 | 12 | 13 | 14 | 15 | 16 | 17 | 18 | 19 | 20 | 21 | 22 | 23 | 24 | 25 | 26 | 27 | 28 | 29 | 30 | | April |
| January | 6 | 7 | 8 | 9 | 10 | 11 | 12 | 13 | 14 | 15 | 16 | 17 | 18 | 19 | 20 | 21 | 22 | 23 | 24 | 25 | 26 | 27 | 28 | 29 | 30 | 31 | 1 | 2 | 3 | 4 | | February |
| May | 1 | 2 | 3 | 4 | 5 | 6 | 7 | 8 | 9 | 10 | 11 | 12 | 13 | 14 | 15 | 16 | 17 | 18 | 19 | 20 | 21 | 22 | 23 | 24 | 25 | 26 | 27 | 28 | 29 | 30 | 31 | May |
| February | 5 | 6 | 7 | 8 | 9 | 10 | 11 | 12 | 13 | 14 | 15 | 16 | 17 | 18 | 19 | 20 | 21 | 22 | 23 | 24 | 25 | 26 | 27 | 28 | 1 | 2 | 3 | 4 | 5 | 6 | 7 | March |
| June | 1 | 2 | 3 | 4 | 5 | 6 | 7 | 8 | 9 | 10 | 11 | 12 | 13 | 14 | 15 | 16 | 17 | 18 | 19 | 20 | 21 | 22 | 23 | 24 | 25 | 26 | 27 | 28 | 29 | 30 | | June |
| March | 8 | 9 | 10 | 11 | 12 | 13 | 14 | 15 | 16 | 17 | 18 | 19 | 20 | 21 | 22 | 23 | 24 | 25 | 26 | 27 | 28 | 29 | 30 | 31 | 1 | 2 | 3 | 4 | 5 | 6 | | April |
| July | 1 | 2 | 3 | 4 | 5 | 6 | 7 | 8 | 9 | 10 | 11 | 12 | 13 | 14 | 15 | 16 | 17 | 18 | 19 | 20 | 21 | 22 | 23 | 24 | 25 | 26 | 27 | 28 | 29 | 30 | 31 | July |
| April | 7 | 8 | 9 | 10 | 11 | 12 | 13 | 14 | 15 | 16 | 17 | 18 | 19 | 20 | 21 | 22 | 23 | 24 | 25 | 26 | 27 | 28 | 29 | 30 | 1 | 2 | 3 | 4 | 5 | 6 | 7 | May |
| August | 1 | 2 | 3 | 4 | 5 | 6 | 7 | 8 | 9 | 10 | 11 | 12 | 13 | 14 | 15 | 16 | 17 | 18 | 19 | 20 | 21 | 22 | 23 | 24 | 25 | 26 | 27 | 28 | 29 | 30 | 31 | August |
| May | 8 | 9 | 10 | 11 | 12 | 13 | 14 | 15 | 16 | 17 | 18 | 19 | 20 | 21 | 22 | 23 | 24 | 25 | 26 | 27 | 28 | 29 | 30 | 31 | 1 | 2 | 3 | 4 | 5 | 6 | 7 | June |
| September | 1 | 2 | 3 | 4 | 5 | 6 | 7 | 8 | 9 | 10 | 11 | 12 | 13 | 14 | 15 | 16 | 17 | 18 | 19 | 20 | 21 | 22 | 23 | 24 | 25 | 26 | 27 | 28 | 29 | 30 | | September |
| June | 8 | 9 | 10 | 11 | 12 | 13 | 14 | 15 | 16 | 17 | 18 | 19 | 20 | 21 | 22 | 23 | 24 | 25 | 26 | 27 | 28 | 29 | 30 | 1 | 2 | 3 | 4 | 5 | 6 | 7 | | July |
| October | 1 | 2 | 3 | 4 | 5 | 6 | 7 | 8 | 9 | 10 | 11 | 12 | 13 | 14 | 15 | 16 | 17 | 18 | 19 | 20 | 21 | 22 | 23 | 24 | 25 | 26 | 27 | 28 | 29 | 30 | 31 | October |
| July | 8 | 9 | 10 | 11 | 12 | 13 | 14 | 15 | 16 | 17 | 18 | 19 | 20 | 21 | 22 | 23 | 24 | 25 | 26 | 27 | 28 | 29 | 30 | 31 | 1 | 2 | 3 | 4 | 5 | 6 | 7 | August |
| November | 1 | 2 | 3 | 4 | 5 | 6 | 7 | 8 | 9 | 10 | 11 | 12 | 13 | 14 | 15 | 16 | 17 | 18 | 19 | 20 | 21 | 22 | 23 | 24 | 25 | 26 | 27 | 28 | 29 | 30 | | November |
| August | 8 | 9 | 10 | 11 | 12 | 13 | 14 | 15 | 16 | 17 | 18 | 19 | 20 | 21 | 22 | 23 | 24 | 25 | 26 | 27 | 28 | 29 | 30 | 31 | 1 | 2 | 3 | 4 | 5 | 6 | | September |
| December | 1 | 2 | 3 | 4 | 5 | 6 | 7 | 8 | 9 | 10 | 11 | 12 | 13 | 14 | 15 | 16 | 17 | 18 | 19 | 20 | 21 | 22 | 23 | 24 | 25 | 26 | 27 | 28 | 29 | 30 | 31 | December |
| September | 7 | 8 | 9 | 10 | 11 | 12 | 13 | 14 | 15 | 16 | 17 | 18 | 19 | 20 | 21 | 22 | 23 | 24 | 25 | 26 | 27 | 28 | 29 | 30 | 1 | 2 | 3 | 4 | 5 | 6 | 7 | October |

Find the first day of your last period on the pink band. The date on the lighter tint below is your estimated date of delivery (EDD).

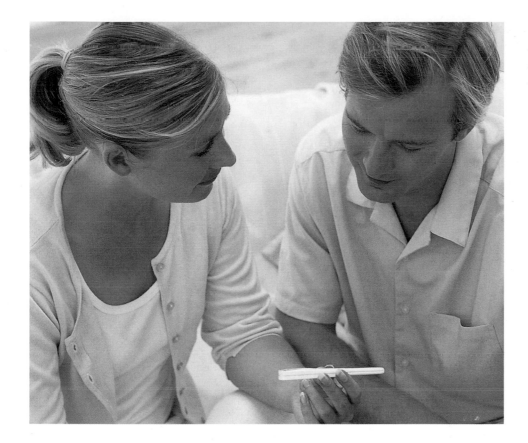

usually shown as a coloured line in the window of the testing strip. The colour may be quite faint, particularly if you are doing the test early on. However, this still counts as a positive result.

The amount of HCG in a woman's body doubles every two or three days during the first six weeks of pregnancy. If a test is negative but your period still does not start, it is worth repeating the test in another two or three days. If the second result is also negative, you are probably not pregnant. See your family doctor for confirmation if you are still unsure.

For optimum results, it can be helpful to do a pregnancy test early in the morning, when HCG is present in its greatest concentrations. However, most modern tests are very sensitive, and they should give an accurate reading at any time of day. You can do the test on the day that your period is due.

### How reliable are pregnancy tests?

Pregnancy tests are extremely reliable – if you get a positive result you are almost certainly pregnant. However sometimes women do the test wrongly or read the result incorrectly. Very occasionally the test fails to work properly or there is not enough HCG to show a positive result. If you are unsure about a result, you can ask your doctor to do a test for you: you will need to provide a urine sample while you are at the surgery.

Finding out that you are not pregnant can be be very disappointing. It is important for you and your partner to take some time to recover from the disappointment and to talk about how you both feel.

### A POSITIVE RESULT

If the result of your test is positive, make an appointment to see your doctor two or three weeks later – when you are about eight weeks pregnant. If you are on any medication, see your doctor sooner – the medication may need to be adjusted to ensure that it does not interfere with the healthy development of your baby.

### What a doctor will do

Your doctor will confirm the pregnancy by doing another pregnancy test. He or she will check that you are taking folic acid and will also ask you about your general health.

You may be offered an ultrasound scan to date the pregnancy if you are not sure when your last period started. A scan through the abdominal wall will show the baby's heartbeat at seven weeks from the last period, so long as you are not overweight. If you are overweight or if the pregnancy is less than seven weeks, a scan through the vagina may be recommended. A vaginal scan can feel slightly uncomfortable, but it does not increase the risk of miscarriage nor does it cause any harm to the baby.

If you have symptoms such as bleeding or pelvic discomfort, a vaginal scan may be done to check that the pregnancy has not established itself outside the uterus (an ectopic pregnancy). This is important because an ectopic pregnancy can be life-threatening if left untreated.

# Early development

By the fourth week of its life, your developing baby is showing the first beginnings of the human form that will develop over the months to come. The sex of your child, the colour of its hair and eyes, its build and potential height, and other genetic characteristics are already decided. The embryo is firmly embedded in the wall of your uterus. Soon, he or she will be floating in a protective sac of warm amniotic fluid.

At this stage, the tiny embryo consists of three layers of tissues, which will develop into different parts of the body. The outer layer of tissue (known as the ectoderm) will grow into the baby's skin and nervous system, as well as its ears and eyes. The middle layer (called the mesoderm) will form the cartilage, bones, connective tissues, muscles and the circulatory system, which includes the heart, the kidneys and the sex organs. The inner layer (the endoderm) will develop into your baby's intestinal tract and digestive system, the lungs and the bladder.

### A CRUCIAL TIME

Many vital tissues and organs form between the fourth and eighth week, making this the most important period in the development of the baby. A harmful substance or an infection is more likely to cause a serious problem at

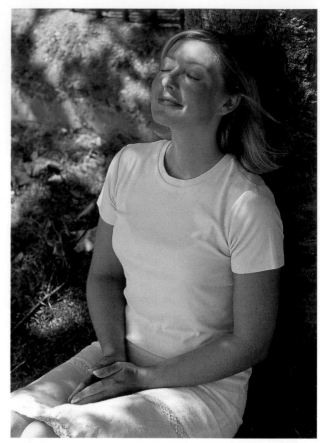

*Your baby develops rapidly during the first few weeks of pregnancy, which is why women tend to feel so tired in the first trimester. To help your baby thrive, you need plenty of rest and early nights, as well as fresh air, regular exercise and a healthy diet.*

this stage rather than later in the pregnancy, when the baby's organs are in place. This is why it is so important for women to look after their general health when they are trying to conceive – because they could already be carrying a baby and not be aware of it.

### Weeks 5–8

Between the fourth and fifth week of its life, the embryo more than doubles in size. By week five, it measures 5-6mm (about ¼in) in length. Despite its tiny size, it has the beginnings of a brain and spinal cord. This develops

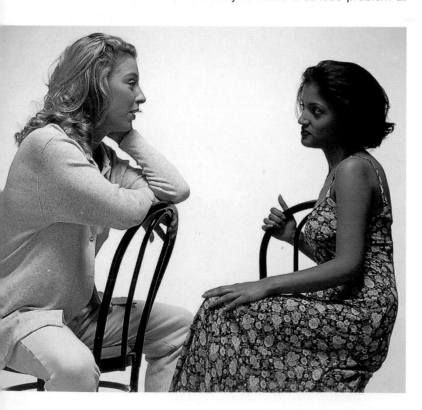

*As soon as you know that you have conceived, your pregnancy may dominate your thoughts. Confiding in a close friend allows you to share your joy and also to voice any mixed feelings or anxieties.*

## EARLY DEVELOPMENT OF THE EMBRYO

Your baby's life starts from the moment that the sperm penetrates the egg – conception. At this point the egg is still in the Fallopian tube, but it will make its way to the uterus over the next few days. As it journeys towards the uterus, the fertilized egg is undergoing the first stages of its development.

### WEEK 1
### FERTILIZATION

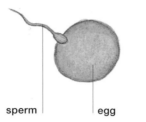

sperm | egg

*Conception occurs when a sperm fertilizes the egg in the Fallopian tube. It will take four days for the fertilized egg to make its way to the uterus.*

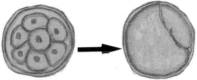

### WEEK 2
### CELL DIVISION

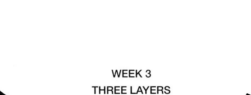

ball of eight cells | blastocyst

*The fertilized egg divides again and again, forming a ball of cells. Eventually, there is a mass of 150 cells, arranged in two sections: the outer cells will develop into the placenta and amniotic sac, while the inner cells become the baby. The blastocyst, as it is now known, attaches itself to the uterus lining.*

### WEEK 3
### THREE LAYERS

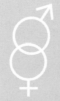

*The inner cells are in three layers. The outer layer will become the baby's skin and nerves; the middle one will be the muscles, heart and skeleton; and the inner one develops into other organs.*

### WEEK 4 +
### DEVELOPING EMBRYO

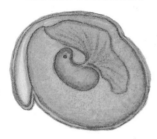

*The tiny embryo begins to take shape. Its brain and spinal cord are starting to develop, and its heart is beating. It is attached to the placenta by a tiny stalk, which will develop into the umbilical cord.*

from the neural tube, which has started to form. At this stage, the baby's heart has already started to beat, although it will not be detectable by ultrasound for another week or two. The heart has only two chambers rather than the four that will develop within another week or so.

The embryo is connected to the developing placenta by a thin stalk, which is the rudimentary beginning of the umbilical cord. Blood vessels are already forming here. From this lifeline, the baby will derive essential nutrients and oxygen, which are needed for its healthy development and growth. At this early stage the placenta is larger than the embryo.

### WHAT THE DOCTORS SAY

Medically, your growing baby is known as an embryo until the eighth week of pregnancy, when all the internal organs are formed. It is then known as a fetus until the delivery.

Medical terms can sound baffling. Always ask about unfamiliar terms and abbreviations that you do not understand. Your doctors and midwife should be happy to explain what they mean.

# Development from six weeks

The embryo develops rapidly from the sixth to eighth week of pregnancy. It passes through a number of phases that some theorists believe resemble the stages of human evolution – from "tadpole" through a fish-like stage to primitive mammal and finally a tiny human being.

### Week 6
During the sixth week, the baby's head forms, rapidly followed by the chest and abdominal cavities. Its rudimentary brain is completed and a spinal column, as well as a spinal cord, is properly formed. The circulation is about to begin functioning. The embryo's heart is now beating steadily, much faster than your own. The stomach is forming, the kidneys are maturing and the liver has grown so much that it almost fills the entire abdominal cavity.

It is also in the sixth week that the baby's face starts to take shape. This is a process that will take several more weeks to complete. Small depressions are appearing where the eyes and ears will be situated. The mouth and jaw are beginning to develop. The embryo is now, incredibly, 10,000 times larger than the fertilized cell from which it originated.

### Week 7
The kidneys and lungs start to develop and the head continues to grow, forming a more recognizably human shape. The buds that will form arms and legs are apparent.

### Week 8
All the internal organs are now formed, although they will continue to mature. The baby now measures 2.5cm (1in) in length. Doctors will now start referring to it as a fetus.

### Weeks 10–11
The baby is moving about a great deal, although you will not yet be able to feel this. The fingers and toes are forming, but are still joined by webs of skin. The facial features are more distinct, and the baby now has eyes.

---

### EARLY DEVELOPMENT, WEEKS 6–13
By week 7, the embryo can be seen on an ultrasound scan. The tiny heart is beating, and the major organs have started to develop. By week 12 or 13, the embryo is a tiny recognizable human with facial features.

**6 WEEKS**

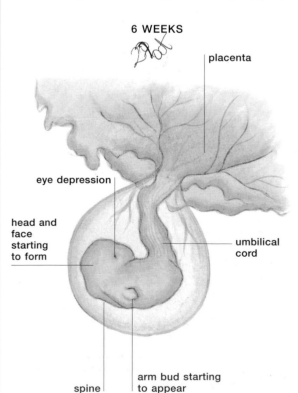

placenta

eye depression

head and face starting to form

umbilical cord

spine

arm bud starting to appear

**7–8 WEEKS**

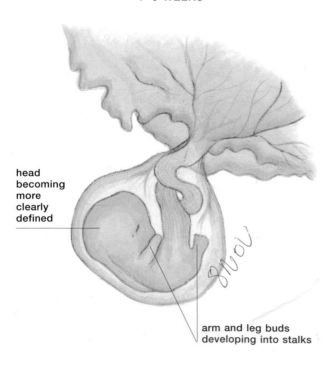

head becoming more clearly defined

arm and leg buds developing into stalks

### Weeks 12–13

The external genitals have formed and all facial features are in place. Your baby measures about 7.5cm (3in) in length (roughly the size of an avocado). The muscles are getting stronger, so movements are more vigorous.

### SEEING YOUR BABY

Ultrasound enables you to see your baby while it is in the uterus. Most people find this a very moving experience, and it can help to strengthen your feelings of connection with your developing baby.

An ultrasound is invaluable in determining the definite existence of a pregnancy as well as the age of the embryo or fetus. You will be offered an early scan to date the pregnancy if you do not know the day of your last period. Otherwise, most women have their first scan at 10–12 weeks. This scan is used to confirm that the baby is able to develop – in medical terms, whether the fetus is viable. The scan can also identify the existence of a multiple pregnancy, so you will know early on if you are carrying twins, triplets or more.

Another scan is usually carried out at about 18 weeks. This scan is used to identify any developmental and structural abnormalities that may not have been apparent at an earlier stage of the pregnancy.

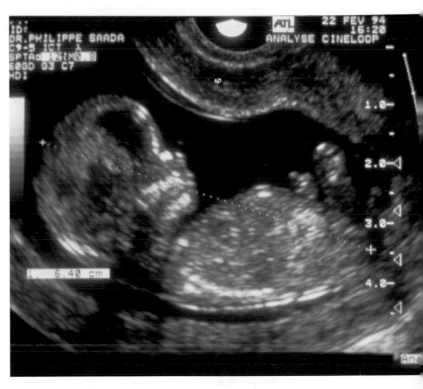

*This is what your baby will look like 12 weeks into your pregnancy – you can see the face at the upper left of the picture. The baby weighs about 45g (1½oz).*

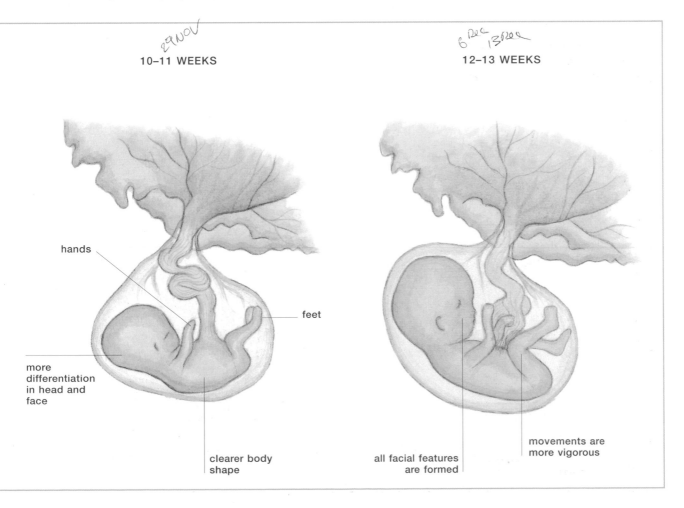

**10–11 WEEKS**

hands

more differentiation in head and face

feet

clearer body shape

**12–13 WEEKS**

all facial features are formed

movements are more vigorous

# How your body is changing

Your baby grows rapidly during the first three months of pregnancy, and your body changes at the same time. However, most of these developments will go unnoticed by anyone except you and, to a lesser extent, your partner. Many women find it hard to believe that they look much the same as normal, but they do.

Your uterus grows to accommodate the developing baby, but by the end of the first trimester it is still no bigger than an avocado pear. Few people will see any difference in your outward appearance. However, when you are naked, you and your partner may notice that your breasts are fuller, and that your nipples have increased in size and darkened. Some women do fill out a little.

The most noticeable effects of your pregnancy, though, will be in the way you feel rather than in the way that you look. Your breasts may tingle. You may experience a feeling of fullness in your abdomen. You are likely to want to pass water more frequently, and you may feel nauseous some or perhaps all of the time. You will probably feel alternately anxious and excited as you come to terms with the fact that you are pregnant.

## FATIGUE

The rapid development rate of the baby in the first weeks of pregnancy is bound to make you feel tired. To help yourself to cope – and to ensure that your baby thrives – you need early nights, regular exercise and a good, healthy diet. Some women feel energized during early

### MEETING YOUR NEEDS
Your body will undergo various changes in the first trimester and you will almost certainly need extra sleep. You may also benefit from doing some of the following:
- Take a rest in the afternoon.
- Drink lots of fruit and vegetable juices.
- Go for a short walk every morning before you start work.
- Swim at lunchtime or after work, two or three times a week.
- Avoid doing any everyday tasks that are not vitally important – for example, ironing or dusting. Ask your partner or friends for help when you need it.
- Wear flat, comfortable shoes.
- Go to bed an hour earlier every night – read in bed for a bit if you don't feel sleepy immediately.
- Treat yourself to an aromatherapy massage or acupuncture session (always seek professional advice about such treatments).
- Buy some relaxing herbal bath preparations and pamper yourself.
- Show your partner that you love, respect and desire him.

pregnancy, but most feel very tired in a way that feels new. You may feel an overwhelming desire to nap in the afternoon, or to get to bed much earlier than usual. The best way to deal with this is to give in to it – rest as much as you can.

## MORNING SICKNESS

Some women sail through their pregnancies without having any nausea, but most experience at least some morning sickness. There are various theories about why this nausea occurs, and some doctors maintain that it is purely psychological. However, most experts think that it is connected to the increased level of hormones circulating in the blood. Morning sickness most commonly affects women in the morning – hence its

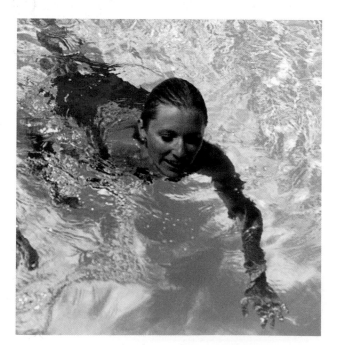

*Swimming – say, two or three times a week – is one of the best forms of exercise in pregnancy. It works all your muscles, and increases flexibility and stamina.*

> **"** Your baby grows rapidly during the first three months, and your body changes at the same time. Most of these developments will go unnoticed. **"**

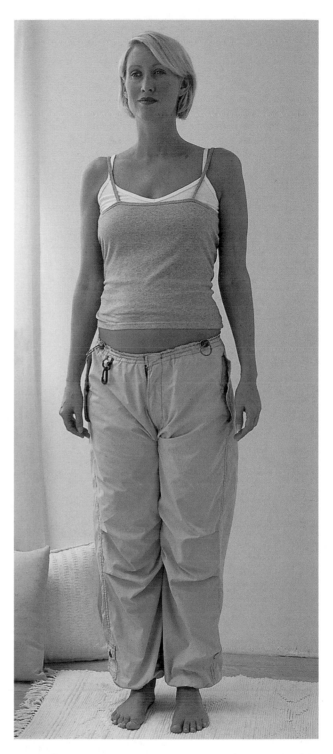

name – but it can also occur at other times of day. Some women feel nauseous all day for the first few weeks. Morning sickness usually starts during the sixth week and continues until the twelfth or fourteenth. However, it sometimes continues throughout pregnancy.

Eating little and often can be helpful, and it is usually best to eat something to raise your blood sugar levels before you get up in the morning. A dry biscuit or piece of toast is ideal. Many women find drinking ginger tea or sucking on a piece of raw ginger can help. You should also make sure you drink plenty of fluids, particularly if you are vomiting.

Morning sickness may be exacerbated by kitchen smells, tobacco smoke and alcohol, so these should be avoided. It is not uncommon to notice flecks of blood in the vomit. This is because repeated vomiting may cause breakage of tiny blood vessels in the throat or gullet. The blood vessels will heal by themselves so there is no need to be alarmed by this. However, if your sickness is very severe, tell your doctor.

## URINATION

One of the earliest signs of pregnancy is an increased frequency in urination. This is known medically as micturition. Some women notice they are passing water more often as early as one week after conception. The increase is due partly to the growing uterus pressing against the nearby bladder, and partly because alterations in hormone levels lead to changes in muscle tone. The increase in frequency of urination is often particularly pronounced in the first nine weeks. After this, the uterus tends to moves upwards, which relieves the pressure on the bladder until much later in the pregnancy.

Some women find that they need to pass water more often throughout their whole pregnancy. It is also quite common to pass a small amount of urine when you laugh or cough. Wearing well-fitting briefs with a light sanitary towel or incontinence pad will help.

*You will soon start to see subtle changes in your body shape as your baby grows and your uterus increases in size to accommodate him or her.*

## TENDER BREASTS

Your breasts may feel heavy and tender, and they often increase in size early on so it is worth investing in a new bra. Your nipples may feel sore and sensitive. They are likely to become harder and may darken in colour. Small white spots may become more pronounced. Breast tenderness is usually relieved after the eighth week.

## TASTE

Pregnant women often report experiencing a strange metallic taste in the mouth. You may also develop new preferences for certain foods and drinks, and go off others – particularly coffee, alcohol and fried foods. Try to resist any cravings for sugary or high-fat snacks since these are high in calories but low in nutrients.

# Emotional changes

The first few months of pregnancy are a time when you and your partner will be discussing all sorts of practical as well as emotional issues. For example, should you stay in the same home or should you move somewhere bigger or closer to family? If you are staying put, do you need to make changes? Will you want to start decorating a nursery?

You need to consider whether you tell close family and friends straight away, or whether you keep the news to yourselves for a few weeks. Keeping quiet can give you a precious opportunity to enjoy and look forward to this very special journey together. Many couples wait until they are past the twelfth week, and they know that the pregnancy is well established, before sharing the news.

## FEELING ANXIOUS

Almost everyone experiences anxiety at some stage of their pregnancy, and most women find that different worries crop up throughout. It is very common to have underlying fears about the health of the baby, particularly before you have gone through any of the antenatal tests. Many women feel anxious about how they will cope with the pregnancy, and how they will deal with the labour and delivery. In addition, couples often doubt their ability to be

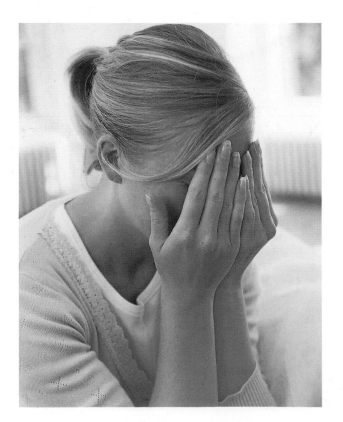

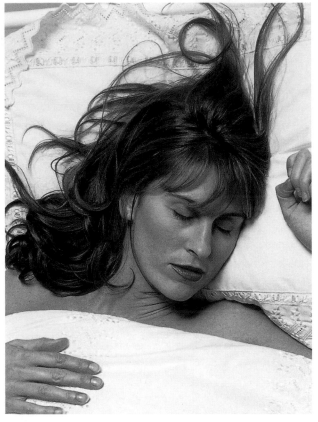

*Most pregnant women find that they want to sleep more; dreams can be very important now, allowing your mind to adapt to the profound life changes ahead.*

good parents and worry about how they will cope with all the practicalities of caring for a child. Concern about the impact that a child will have on your financial situation, sexual relationship, careers and social lives can all surface during pregnancy.

It is important to keep a sense of perspective, and to realize that doubts and worries are perfectly normal. After all, you are embarking on a life-changing event. However, if anxiety starts to dominate your thinking, it can be helpful to confide in a close friend or relative who has had a child, or to talk to your midwife.

You may also experience strange dreams about giving birth or becoming a mother. These dreams reflect the natural anxiety that you feel, and they are also a way of preparing psychologically for the new role ahead of you.

*Fluctuating hormone levels may play havoc with your emotions and stability. Get plenty of rest and recognize any volatility for the biological phenomenon that it is.*

## COMMUNICATING WITH YOUR BABY

Some women find that they do not experience a sense of connection with their baby until later in their pregnancy – and occasionally only after the birth. However, many women feel a bond with the growing baby early on, perhaps as soon as they know they are pregnant. This can be a very special feeling; suddenly the most important thing in the world is the health and well-being of the tiny baby inside you.

Fathers often do not feel a sense of bonding in the first months, when there is little outward sign of the baby's presence. This is understandable, but many women find it hard to accept their partner is not quite so fascinated with the pregnancy as they are. Both partners may need to exercise some tolerance about the different ways that they react to the pregnancy.

It usually helps if the father gets involved right from the start. Ideally he will attend any scans so that he can see the baby on screen. Some men like to talk to the baby through the mother's abdomen. Stroking the mother's

*"Suddenly the most important thing in the world is the health and well-being of the tiny baby inside you."*

belly or playing music to the baby can also help fathers to feel more connected with the life they have created.

Nobody knows how much unborn babies can hear or feel in the uterus, but some research shows that they learn to recognize their parents' voices before they are born. The ears are formed by the seventh week, and it is known that external sounds filter through. Researchers have now found that unborn babies can also distinguish different intonation patterns – so they may be able to recognize the speech sounds you and your partner make.

*Communicating with your baby can help you and your partner to bond with your unborn child, long before he or she comes into the world to be part of your family.*

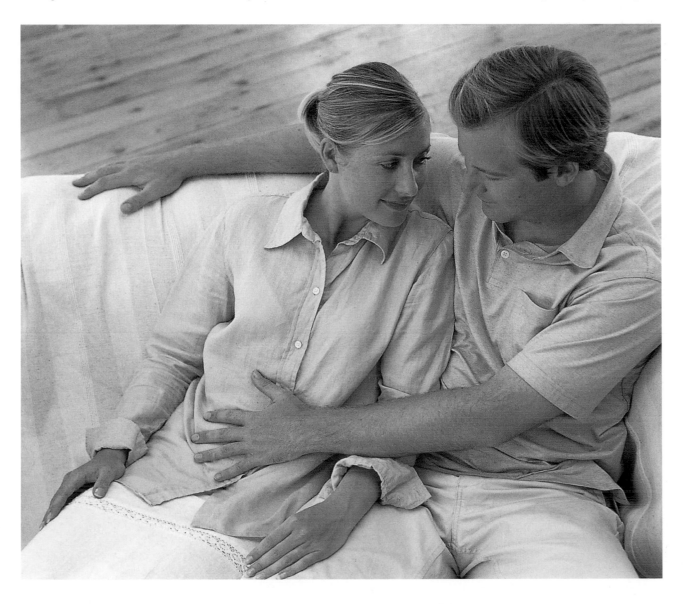

# Pregnancy and eating

Make sure that you establish healthy eating patterns in the first trimester, because for all of your pregnancy, and longer if you are breastfeeding, your baby depends on you for its water and essential nutrients. Getting into good habits also means that you will be eating well when your child is born, helping you to cope with the demands of motherhood, and you can then go on to share your healthy eating patterns with your child. Follow these simple rules for a sensible and achievable approach to eating:

- Eat a balanced diet, including food from each of the main food groups every day.
- Eat five helpings of fruit and vegetables every day.
- Minimize your intake of animal fats and sugars.
- Drink at least eight glasses of water every day.
- Have regular meals.
- Choose natural unprocessed foods wherever possible.
- Avoid a few potentially harmful foods (see pages 24–5).

The five main food groups are as follows:

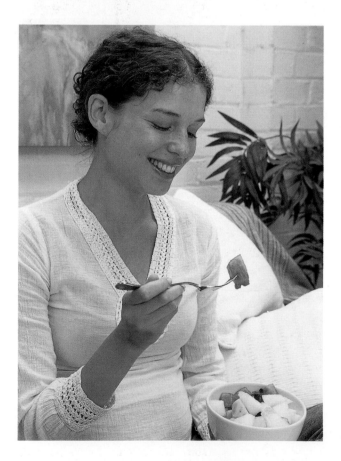

*When pregnant, eating small meals at frequent intervals can ease morning sickness, heartburn and indigestion.*

## GROUP 1: BREADS AND OTHER CEREALS

These are excellent sources of carbohydrate, which gives us energy, and fibre, which helps keep the digestive tract healthy. They also supply B vitamins, calcium and iron. Eat whole grains, such as wholemeal bread and pasta and brown rice, wherever possible.

## GROUP 2: FRUIT AND VEGETABLES

Fruits and vegetables contain a wide range of vitamins and minerals, have almost no fat and are a good source of fibre. Eat them raw or lightly cooked to obtain maximum nutritional value.

## GROUP 3: MEAT, FISH AND ALTERNATIVES

Beef, lamb, pork and bacon are good protein sources, needed for vital functions such as cell-repair. They also provide minerals such as iron and zinc, and B vitamins. Opt for lean cuts and trim off fat. Fish and poultry also provide protein. Oily fish such as mackerel, salmon and sardines are rich in nutritious fish oils; try to eat two portions a week. Grill, steam, microwave or bake fish rather than deep-frying it.

Nuts, peas, lentils, soya and pulses contain protein but, unlike meat or fish, do not have all the essential amino acids needed for growth. To redress this, serve them with plant foods and whole grains such as wholemeal bread.

## GROUP 4: MILK AND OTHER DAIRY PRODUCTS

Dairy produce such as eggs, cheese, milk and milk products provide calcium, which builds teeth and bones, and some protein. Pregnant women need lots of calcium to build their baby's skeleton. It is generally better to choose low-fat products.

## GROUP 5: FAT AND SUGAR

We need some fat in our diet. There are two main types: saturated and unsaturated. Saturated fats, such as butter and lard, can increase blood cholesterol and with it the risk of heart disease. The two forms of unsaturated fat – monounsaturated and polyunsaturated – are better for you and may also lower cholesterol levels. Monounsaturated fats include olive oil and avocado; polyunsaturated fats include most vegetable oils, fish oil and nuts. Pick low-fat dairy products and use olive oil in place of butter.

Sugary foods provide a short-term energy boost, but little nutritional value. Eat sparingly, if at all.

## IMPORTANT NUTRITIONAL REQUIREMENTS

It is especially important during pregnancy to have sufficient protein, iron, calcium, folic acid and fibre.

## PROTEIN

You need 60–100g (2¼–3¾oz) protein per day, and high-protein foods should constitute about 25 per cent of your diet. Good sources include vegetables, lean meat, chicken, fish, eggs, skimmed milk, nuts, cheese, dried peas, beans and grains.

## IRON

Pregnancy greatly increases the volume of blood in a mother's body. This means that extra iron is needed to make haemoglobin, the oxygen-carrying pigment in red blood cells. The more haemoglobin that blood contains, the more oxygen it can carry to the various tissues, including the placenta, keeping the organs of the mother and baby healthy and helping to prevent the mother from becoming over-tired. The recommended daily amount (RDA) of iron required in pregnancy is 30mg. The need for iron increases particularly in the second and third trimesters.

Good sources of iron include red meat, dark poultry meat, breads, cereals, dried peas and beans, broccoli and green leafy vegetables. Vitamin C helps the body to absorb iron from other, plant-based sources more efficiently, so it is a good idea to have a glass of orange juice or a tomato salad with meals. Another simple way of increasing iron intake is to use iron pans when cooking.

Pregnant women used to be given iron tablets as a matter of course. This should not be necessary so long as you eat a good diet with sufficient iron-rich foods (although it may be necessary if you are expecting two or more babies). If you are worried about iron intake, or feel tired for no apparent reason, see a doctor. A simple blood test will determine if you are deficient (anaemic). It can be

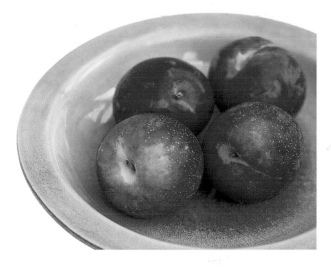

*Plums and other fruits provide you with beneficial vitamins and help to combat constipation. They can also give you a quick boost when you feel tired.*

hard to get enough iron if you do not eat red meat, so vegetarians and vegans will often be advised to take iron supplements.

## CALCIUM

You need about 1,200mg of this each day in pregnancy. Good sources include milk, all other dairy products and green vegetables. A growing baby needs calcium to build strong bones and teeth and will take calcium from your bones and teeth if you do not eat enough of it. Your body absorbs calcium more efficiently during pregnancy, and your baby is unlikely to go short, although this may not leave you enough for your own requirements.

You should make sure that you take plenty of calcium-rich foods throughout your pregnancy. You need the equivalent of 600ml (1 pint) milk a day. A small pot of yogurt or 25g (1oz) hard cheese contain as much calcium as about 200ml (⅓ pint) milk. Vegans and women who never drink milk, because they are allergic to it or don't like it, may need calcium supplements. If you eat well, 600mg should be enough, but 1,200mg may be advised in some cases.

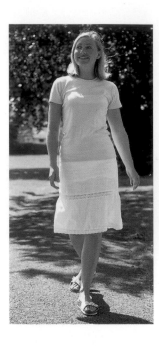

*Take a short walk every day so that you receive exposure to sunlight. This enables the body to manufacture vitamin D, which in turn aids the absorption of calcium.*

### Calcium and vitamin D

You also need vitamin D to help your body to absorb and process calcium properly. This vital vitamin is found in milk, butter and eggs. More importantly, however, the body can manufacture its own vitamin D if it is exposed to the sun. You should therefore try to take a short walk outdoors each day in order to expose your face, hands and arms to daylight.

### FOLIC ACID

An essential B vitamin, folic acid (folate) cannot be produced by the body, so it must be obtained either through diet or supplements. Your daily folic acid requirement increases considerably in pregnancy, to 400mcg. Make sure that you receive enough by taking a daily supplement of 400mcg. You should also try to eat at least one dark green vegetable and two to three servings of fruit a day. Sprinkling wheatgerm onto food and not overcooking it also help maximize your folic acid intake – overcooking food destroys any folic acid content.

### What folic acid does

Folic acid intake is especially important during the first 12 weeks of pregnancy, as it helps the baby's spine and brain to develop properly. Folic acid can help protect an unborn baby from developing spina bifida (an abnormal development of the spinal cord) and anencephaly (absence of most of the brain). Infants born with anencephaly die shortly after birth, and babies with spina bifida are born with partial or total paralysis.

### FIBRE

Fibre is an indigestible substance that we get from nuts, cereals, fruit and vegetables, and is vital for speeding up the passage of waste products through the bowel and

removing toxins. Constipation is common during pregnancy, when bowel movements slow down, but plenty of fibre-rich food and water help to prevent this. It can also be helpful to avoid bananas, hard-boiled eggs, Brussels sprouts and red meat for a few days.

### ZINC

You also need zinc to help the baby develop – there is evidence to suggest that an inadequate intake is linked to low birthweight. Make sure that you are eating enough zinc-rich foods; the body's levels of zinc can fall by as much as 30 per cent during pregnancy.

### PROTECTING YOUR BABY

The baby takes the nutrients it needs from the mother's bloodstream through the placenta. Poor intake of one or more essential nutrients during critical periods in an organ's growth can alter the structure, size and functions of that organ. Mothers who eat an excessive amount and who consume a diet high in saturated fat could be putting their unborn babies at greater risk of heart disease, diabetes and high blood pressure later in life.

### HOW MUCH SHOULD YOU EAT?

Because a developing baby's health is affected by what the mother eats, mothers-to-be were traditionally advised to 'eat for two'. Experts no longer regard this as sensible advice, but that is not to say that the opposite is true. Some women eat too little during pregnancy, to keep their weight down. The amount of food that you need to eat does not increase that much during pregnancy. However,

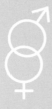

**RATE OF WEIGHT GAIN**
The following is a rough guide to the rate of weight gain through a normal pregnancy:

| | |
|---|---|
| 0–12 weeks | 10 per cent |
| 13–20 weeks | 25 per cent |
| 21–28 weeks | 45 per cent |
| 29–36 weeks | 20 per cent |
| 37–40 weeks | 0 per cent |

make sure that you are eating enough to receive the essential nutrients and remember that undereating can lead to more difficult labours and underweight babies and may increase the risk of miscarriage and death around the time of delivery. Heavier babies are often healthier and better able to resist common childhood illnesses. However, pregnant women who gain an excessive amount are at greater risk of developing diabetes, as are their babies.

## WHY WOMEN GAIN WEIGHT IN PREGNANCY

Women lay down fat early in pregnancy as preparation for milk production and breastfeeding. This fat remains after the birth, but should gradually disappear if you eat well and exercise regularly. Other weight gain comes from the placenta, the fluids around the baby, the baby itself (this accounts for more than half of the total weight gain) and the extra blood produced by pregnant women to support a healthy pregnancy.

Everyone is different and so there are no strict rules about how much weight pregnant women should put on. Most women tend to gain around 9–13.5kg (20–30lb) during pregnancy. However, someone who is already overweight may not need to put on as much weight during her pregnancy as a woman who is underweight. That said, the overweight woman should not try to diet once she knows that she is pregnant.

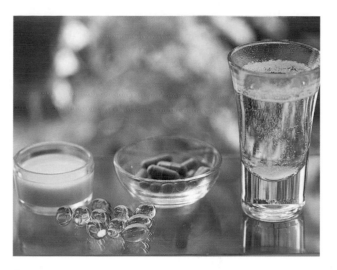

*Supplements come in a number of different forms. Chelated supplements are said to be more rapidly absorbed by the body.*

**DO I NEED SUPPLEMENTS?**
You do need more of certain nutrients when pregnant. For example, your iron requirement almost doubles while your baby is growing. Many experts believe that pregnant women can obtain all the nutrients they need from a healthy, balanced diet. The main exception that applies to all women is folic acid, needed before conception and in early pregnancy in an amount that is difficult to derive from food. Most women should not need to take other supplements, as long as they eat regular, healthy meals, although there are cases where it may be suggested. For example, some women may be advised to start taking supplements such as iron or calcium as the pregnancy progresses.

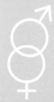

**ESSENTIAL VITAMINS AND MINERALS**
Certain vitamins and minerals are vital for a healthy pregnancy. You may need a higher-than-average daily intake of some nutrients, such as vitamin B1. Use the following list to help you to plan your pregnancy diet:

- **Vitamin A:** 700mcg a day – from fortified milk, eggs, carrots and dark green leafy vegetables.
- **Vitamin B1 or thiamine:** about 1.4mg a day – from enriched breads, cereals, grain products, seeds and nuts.
- **Vitamin B2 or riboflavin:** 1.4mg a day – from meat, dairy produce and cereals.
- **Vitamin B3 or niacin:** from fish, meat, nuts and wholegrains.
- **Vitamin B6 or pyridoxine:** from chicken, fish, soya beans and oats.
- **Vitamin B12 or cobalamin:** from meat, fish, eggs and milk and also from enriched grain products.
- **Vitamin C:** 50mg – from citrus fruit, tomatoes, red and green peppers, broccoli, cauliflower, spinach and strawberries.
- **Vitamin D:** 10mg a day – from milk, eggs, butter and fortified margarine.
- **Vitamin E:** from margarine, vegetable oils, wholegrains and nuts.
- **Magnesium:** 300mg a day – from dairy products, vegetables and meat.
- **Zinc:** 7–15mg a day – from nuts, wholegrains, legumes and eggs.

# Avoiding toxic substances

**P**regnant women should limit their intake of toxic substances. While it may be hard to shut out industrial emissions, for example, you can easily avoid dangers such as smoky atmospheres and certain foods and chemicals.

## FOODS AND DRINKS TO AVOID

The following foods may cause harm to you or your baby and should ideally be avoided completely.

- **Soft, blue-veined and unpasteurized cheese** such as Brie and goat's cheese, due to the risk of listeriosis.
- **Raw or lightly cooked eggs and poultry**, as hens may be infected by salmonella and other bacteria. Eggs and chicken must be well cooked to prevent infection.
- **Raw beef** including steak tartare, rare beef and undercooked beefburgers, regardless of where the meat comes from, because of the risk of BSE.
- **Certain fish**, because they contain mercury, which can harm an unborn baby's developing nervous system. Avoid shark, swordfish and marlin and eat no more than one tuna steak or two medium cans of tuna each week.
- **Shellfish and raw fish**, which carry a higher-than-average risk of food poisoning.
- **Liver**, liver pâté and liver sausage. They are high in vitamin A, which can cause damage to the fetus.
- **Unpasteurized milk**, which may harbour highly harmful bacteria, including salmonella and listeria.

Minimize your intake of the following foods and drinks:

- **Alcohol**, which may impede the uptake of B-vitamins, zinc and iron and harm a fetus.

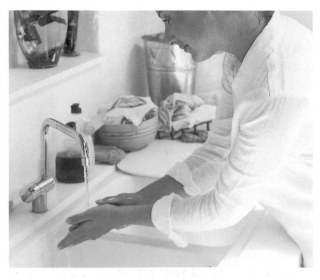

*Be sure to wash your hands with antibacterial soap both before and after handling foods.*

- **Tea and coffee**, whose caffeine content may impede iron uptake. One study found that over 300mg of caffeine a day may be linked with miscarriage, and pregnant women who drank eight or more cups of coffee a day were found to have double the risk of stillbirth as women who drank no coffee. The 300mg caffeine limit is roughly equivalent to: four cups/three mugs of instant coffee; three cups of brewed coffee; six cups of tea; eight cans of regular cola drinks; four cans of energy drinks; two 200g (7oz) chocolate bars.
- **Sugary foods** such as cookies, cakes and other sweet snacks and drinks, which contain few nutrients.
- **Fried foods and junk food**, which are high in unhealthy fats and should be avoided where possible.
- **Salt**, from adding salt to food to eating salty snacks such as crisps (US potato chips). Excess salt increases the risk of high blood pressure, which can be harmful.
- **Convenience foods and takeaway meals**, as these have poor nutrient value. Eat fresh, natural foods.

## PREVENTING FOOD POISONING

Poor food hygiene causes thousands of food poisoning cases every year. Pregnant women must take great care to avoid food poisoning, since there is a real threat to the unborn baby. Food poisoning is usually the result of eating food contaminated by bacteria. These precautions will help prevent bacteria from spreading and multiplying:

- Wash your hands with hot water and an antibacterial soap before and after handling food, especially poultry, raw meat, fish, seafood, salads, vegetables and eggs.
- Wash your hands with hot water and antibacterial soap after handling cats, dogs and other domestic pets.
- Disinfect kitchen surfaces with an antibacterial solution.
- Use plastic (not wooden) chopping boards, disinfected after each use. Use separate boards for cooked and raw foods.
- Fridges should be kept at under 5°C (41°F). Use a fridge thermometer to be sure the temperature is right.
- Store raw foods separately from ready-to-eat and cooked foods (place raw meat and fish on the bottom shelf of the fridge). Always abide by use-by dates.
- Regularly clean taps, telephones and any gadgets in the kitchen, using an antibacterial solution.

### Avoiding listeriosis

Listeriosis is caused by the bacterium *Listeria monocytogenes*. If caught during pregnancy, it can result in miscarriage, stillbirth or severe illness in the baby. High levels of listeria have been found in the following foods, so it is best to avoid them:

- Unpasteurized milk.
- Pâté made from meat, fish or vegetables.
- Mould-ripened and blue-veined cheeses.
- Soft-whip ice cream from ice-cream machines.
- Pre-cooked poultry and cook-chill meals unless thoroughly reheated.
- Prepared salads, unless washed thoroughly.

### Avoiding Campylobacter pylori

The bacterium *Campylobacter pylori* is the chief cause of food poisoning in the UK and the USA – it accounts for over 2.5 million cases in the USA every year. The bacterium is found in raw meat, poultry, wild birds and unpasteurized milk, so pregnant women should avoid raw and lightly cooked eggs and undercooked chicken.

### Avoiding salmonella

Salmonella is a bacterium commonly found in hens. Be sure to cook poultry and eggs thoroughly during pregnancy. Do not eat foods containing raw egg, such as fresh mayonnaise.

### Avoiding toxoplasmosis

Toxoplasmosis is an infection caused by a parasite that can cause miscarriage or damage to the unborn baby. It may be present in soil, so fresh fruit, vegetables and lettuce are all potential sources of infection. They should be thoroughly washed under running water.

### OTHER HAZARDS TO AVOID

We know that some environmental substances, in particular toxins and radiation, may endanger pregnancy. Although currently available research is not clear-cut, it seems sensible to reduce your exposure to hazards wherever you can. Here are some of the things you should avoid in pregnancy.

### X-rays

Having an X-ray exposes you to a tiny dose of radiation. The dose is too small to cause problems for you, but it can sometimes have an adverse effect on a fetus. Always tell your doctor or dentist if you are pregnant, and if possible have any medical or dental investigations carried out before you attempt to conceive. If you had an X-ray before realizing you were pregnant, talk to your doctor. In most cases, there is unlikely to be a problem.

### Other sources of radiation

Computers, VDUs and TVs are sometimes cited as a hazard because they give out small amounts of radiation. However, the general advice is that they do not emit enough radiation to have an effect on pregnancy.

### CHEMICAL PRODUCTS

Certain room deodorizers, furniture polish, oven cleaners, weedkillers and other products may contain poisonous substances. Always read labels carefully, and seek out household cleaning and garden products that are non-toxic and environment-friendly.

Take special care if you are exposed to chemicals at work – for example, if you are a hairdresser or a gardener. Talk to your doctor or midwife about whether or not any substances you come into contact with could be harmful to your pregnancy.

Research on the effect of mobile phones on the brain and nervous system is not yet clear, but it is wise to reduce your use to a minimum and use a hands-free model whenever possible. Do not chat with the mobile held next to your head while in an enclosed area such as a car.

### Cats and kittens

The faeces of kittens and young cats may carry the potentially damaging parasite toxoplasmosis. The faeces are infectious only when kittens or young cats first acquire toxoplasmosis – usually while hunting during their first year. To protect yourself, avoid contact with kittens and young cats wherever possible. Always wear gloves if you have to empty a cat-litter tray, and disinfect it with boiling water for five minutes every day. There may also be toxoplasmosis in the soil, so wear gloves for gardening and wash your hands thoroughly after contact with soil.

### Appliances

Get appliances such as microwave ovens or gas heaters checked to make sure that they are working properly and are not leaking radiation or carbon monoxide.

### Livestock

Do not touch pregnant livestock if you are pregnant. They may carry bacteria that can cause miscarriage.

### Long-haul flights

Sitting in one position for a long period – as when flying – increases your risk of deep vein thrombosis (DVT). In DVT a blood clot forms in the leg or pelvis. This can become detached and travel to the lungs, a condition that can be life-threatening. Pregnant women are at greater risk of developing DVT. To help prevent it, get up every hour or so to move around. At regular intervals in between, flex your wrists and ankles and stretch your neck to left, right and downwards in order to keep freshly oxygenated blood flowing around the body. Drink plenty of water before, during and after the flight and avoid any alcohol.

# Good ways to exercise

The following forms of exercise can be of particular benefit during pregnancy:

- dancing
- swimming
- walking
- t'ai chi
- Pilates
- yoga

If you are not used to exercising, confine yourself to regular walking or swimming in the first three months. Thereafter, it should be fine to try a new form of exercise provided that you have not experienced any bleeding or other problems. Check with your midwife or doctor first, build up your fitness slowly, and do not to overstretch yourself. Seek out a professional instructor who is used to working with pregnant women.

### SWIMMING

A few lengths at your local pool can be remarkably energizing. The water will take the weight of your body so that you can move freely. Swimming helps to improve your suppleness as well as your stamina. It also helps to stimulate blood flow around your body, and thus increases the delivery of oxygen to your growing baby.

You may like to consider taking swimming classes to improve your technique, and to ensure that you are not putting unnecessary strain on your body. The Shaw method is based on Alexander technique, and will help you to use your body in the most efficient way possible. Another great form of water exercise is aqua yoga – literally, yoga in water – and many local pools and leisure clubs offer classes in this.

### WALKING

Like swimming, walking is a great form of exercise when you are pregnant. A brisk walk really helps to stimulate your respiratory and cardiovascular systems, which need to be in good form when you are carrying a baby and in preparation for the birth itself. Walking is also good for encouraging circulation in the legs – thus helping to prevent varicose veins – and it gets you out into the open air, which usually encourages good sleep and relaxation. Cycling offers many of the same benefits.

### DANCE THERAPY

Going to dance classes is usually good fun, and a great way of socializing, making new friends and maintaining fitness at the same time. You will find a number of

## Exercising in water

Doing simple exercises and stretches in water is an especially good idea when you are pregnant because the water is so supportive. The two steps shown below use the water's resistance to help tone your upper

arms, which can accumulate fat during pregnancy. This exercise will also open the chest, helping the heart to work faster as your baby grows, and strengthen the upper body in general, aiding your posture.

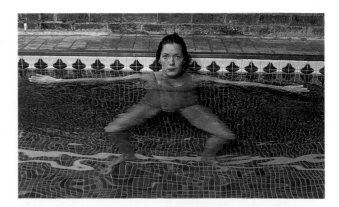

**1** The water should come up to your neck, so stand with your knees slightly bent, if necessary, or kneel if the water is shallow. Now, with both palms touching, stretch your arms right out in front of you.

**2** Turn your hands out and open your arms in a wide, circling movement. Take them as far back as possible, then return to the centre. Repeat several times. Inhale as you stretch out and exhale as you return to the centre.

different dance classes on offer at all kinds of places in your local area, and private classes may also be available – a good way to start if you are self-conscious.

One exciting way of keeping fit during pregnancy could be belly dancing. This gentle, rhythmic exercise promotes muscle strength and stamina, so it can help you to manage pregnancy and labour. Belly dancing originated from a combination of symbolic rituals and sexual display. The undulating movements of the pelvis and abdomen, which involve considerable muscular control, are thought by some to be symbolic of conception and birth. These are usually beneficial during a normal pregnancy, but check with your midwife or doctor first. Look out for classes aimed specifically at pregnant women.

### PILATES

A gentle form of exercise that improves flexibility, strength and stamina, Pilates places a strong emphasis on posture and alignment. Pilates works on both mind and body, so it can induce deep relaxation and a sense of greater control over your body, which may be helpful during labour.

Exercises can be tailored to individual needs, so Pilates can be practised safely throughout pregnancy as long as you already understand the basic techniques and avoid certain postures. Seek advice from an experienced, qualified teacher, and be sure to tell them that you are pregnant. If you are new to Pilates, do not start in the first three months of pregnancy.

### YOGA

Certain types of yoga are widely recommended for pregnancy, particularly the second and third trimesters. Practised regularly, it strengthens muscles, enhances suppleness and improves posture – all of which are helpful during pregnancy and labour. Yoga also involves breathing exercises, which can help with relaxation.

Specific yoga postures, such as squatting, are particularly helpful for pregnant women; others are not suitable and may be harmful. It is therefore best to attend special antenatal yoga classes, or ask your teacher how to adapt the poses. Do not go to general classes if you are new to yoga, particularly in the first trimester.

### T'AI CHI

Sometimes described as 'meditation in motion', t'ai chi is a non-combative martial art that involves moving very slowly through a set routine of postures. You repeat the routine over and over again, producing a flowing, synchronized series of movements.

T'ai chi involves controlled, slow movements, which aim to improve the body's flow of energy. It helps mobilize the joints, improve posture and enhance well-being. T'ai chi aids relaxation and enhances body-awareness. It is generally considered safe in pregnancy.

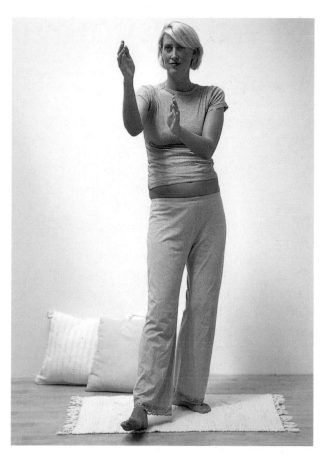

*T'ai chi's flowing, meditative movements will help to enhance your awareness of what is happening to your body and mind during pregnancy.*

### EXERCISING DURING PREGNANCY

You should exercise regularly (ideally for at least 30 minutes, three times a week) in order to work the muscles and circulation, raise energy and endorphin levels and combat stress.

If you have an established exercise routine, it is safe to continue it provided that there are no problems with the pregnancy, but tell any instructors that you are pregnant. However, you may need to reduce the amount or the intensity of any exercise as you must not overexert or exhaust yourself when pregnant (so avoid long periods of aerobic exercise). Do not let yourself become overheated or dehydrated, as this can reduce blood flow and in turn the supply of oxygen to your baby (drink plenty of water as you exercise). If you experience problems with your pregnancy, such as bleeding or abdominal pain, ask your doctor about the advisability of exercising.

In general, it is not a good idea to start a new, unfamiliar form of exercise in the first months of pregnancy. This is because you can easily cause yourself harm if your technique is incorrect.

# Keeping your joints mobile

It is important to keep your body open and flexible, in order to enjoy a pregnancy that is as free as possible from aches and pains, and to help pave the way towards a good, comfortable birth.

Releasing the head, neck and shoulders will help to get you into good posture habits, ease stress and minimize certain kinds of tension headache. It will also help to expand the chest, improving breathing and circulation and so making you feel more energetic and helping to bring plenty of nourishing, oxygen-rich blood to your developing baby. The beauty of the neck and shoulder exercises shown below is that they can be done virtually anywhere, any time, as you sit at your desk at work, watch television or sit on the bus, for example.

## Loosening the joints

Anyone can do the following easy stretches, which will help to keep your joints mobile and flexible. They make a good short loosening-up routine for the morning, and can help you to warm up for more aerobic exercise, such as brisk walking on the spot or cycling. Work very gently and go only as far as feels comfortable to you.

### RELEASING THE HEAD AND NECK

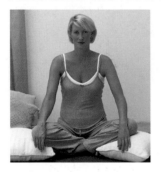 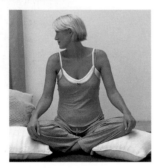 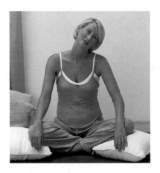 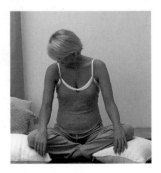

**1** Sit comfortably on the floor, cross-legged or with one leg in front of the other. Place one cushion under your buttocks and another under each knee.

**2** Slowly turn your head to the right and bring it back to the centre. Now turn it slowly to the left. Repeat several times, breathing normally as you do so.

**3** Now slowly drop your head so that your ear is close to your right shoulder. Return it to the centre, then repeat on the left. Repeat several times.

**4** Turn your head to the right, drop your chin close to your chest, then move over to the left. Repeat in the opposite direction. Repeat several times.

### RELEASING THE SHOULDERS

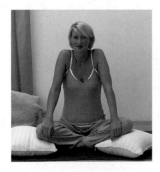 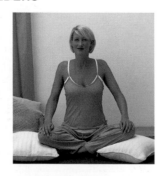 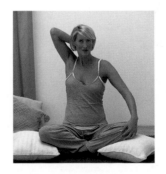 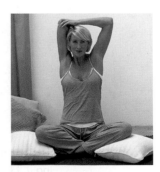

**1** Bring your shoulders upwards and slightly forwards, until they are close to your ears. Keep breathing as you do so.

**2** Then move the shoulders back and down, to make a rotating movement. Repeat this several times.

**3** Raise your right arm, bending the elbow. Drop your forearm down so that you can place your palm in your upper back.

**4** Hold the elbow with the left hand. Relax the shoulders, and hold for a few moments, breathing deeply. Repeat on the left.

Loosening up the spine helps to keep it strong and supple. A flexible spine is the lynchpin of good, upright posture, which can start to suffer with the weight of a growing baby. Correct posture brings these benefits:

- It holds the uterus in the correct position and opens up more space in the abdominal area, so making pregancy more comfortable for both you and your baby and ensuring that the blood supply to the uterus is not constricted.
- It opens up the chest cavity, which becomes more restricted as your baby grows in size, and so improves breathing and circulation, the benefits of which have been covered opposite.

- It makes you feel and look better and minimizes the backache, cramp and sciatica suffered by so many pregnant women.

Loosening up the hips and legs brings vital benefits. The exercise shown below helps to:

- Rest the lower back and legs, which often feel tired and achy during pregnancy.
- Open up your entire pelvic region, exercising and toning the all-important muscles of the pelvic floor area. Well-toned pelvic muscles help to: keep you comfortable when the baby is pressing against the pelvic floor; ease the baby's actual birth; prevent certain post-natal problems.

## RELEASING THE SPINE

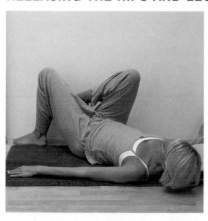

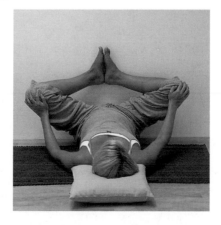

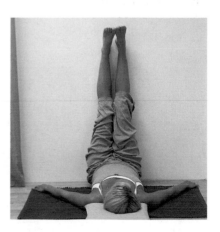

**1** Place your left hand on your right knee, gently turn the upper body and look over your right shoulder.

**2** Drop your shoulders, hold for a few moments, then return to the centre. Keep breathing deeply.

**3** Repeat on the other side. Be very gentle, and take care not to push your body into a strong twist.

## RELEASING THE HIPS AND LEGS

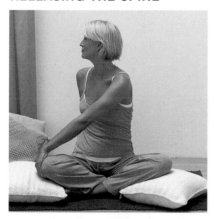

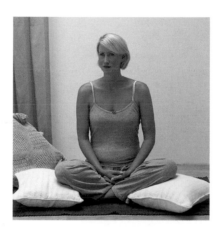

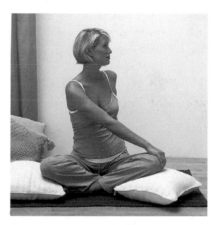

**1** Sit next to a wall, so that the side of your body is facing it. Lie down, moving from your side to your back, and slowly swinging your legs up the wall as you do so. Your buttocks should touch the wall. Rest your head on a cushion and breathe.

**2** Bend your knees, bringing the soles of your feet together. Place your hands on your knees and press gently towards the wall. Hold for a few moments, or longer if you like, then release. Do not force this: your flexibility will improve with practice.

**3** Slide your legs back up the wall. Remain in this posture for a few minutes if you like, breathing deeply and letting any tension drain away. To come up, bend your knees again and then roll on to your side, before getting up slowly.

# Yoga for the first trimester

These easy yoga exercises help to improve the posture, which can be adversely affected during pregnancy. Always take care when practising yoga poses, even simple ones like these. Go only as far as feels comfortable, and keep breathing evenly throughout. Lie down and relax for five minutes afterwards.

## Grounding

Your hips, legs and feet take your weight, while the pelvis helps support the upper body. These important muscle groups can be strengthened by this grounding exercise, which allows your weight to pass through the legs and feet into the ground. Practised regularly, it will help you cope with the growing weight of your baby.

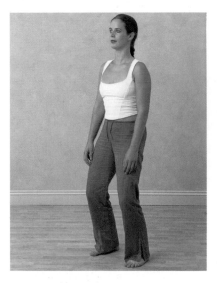

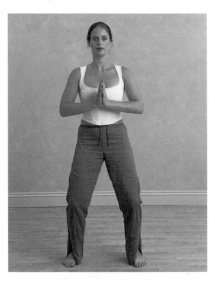

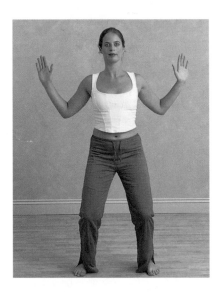

**1** Stand with the feet apart and knees slightly bent. Keep an upright spine, tucking in your chin and tail bone, and keeping the head erect.

**2** Bring your hands into a prayer position. Press your palms firmly together with elbows out to the sides. Do not tense the shoulders.

**3** Now spread your hands wide, keeping your elbows bent and opening up your chest area. Breathe in deeply as you do this.

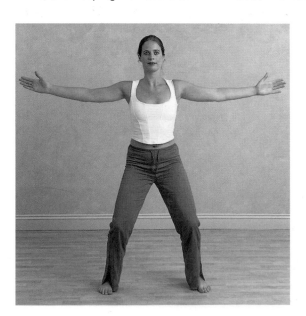

**4** Left: Stretch your arms out to the sides and lower them to your sides, breathing out. Repeat steps 2 to 4 several times.

**5** Right: For a stronger version of this exercise, place one foot on a low chair and bend the other knee. Change legs after a few breaths and repeat with the other foot on the chair.

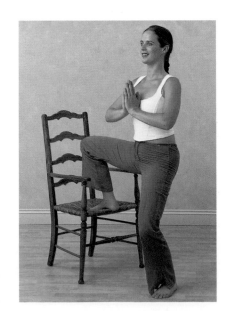

# Standing stretches

By extending up from the hips and through the waist, you create space for the diaphragm, which helps you to take deeper breaths. Gently turn and sway rhythmically as if you are dancing, but do not go into a strong twist.

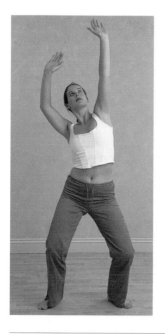

**1** Left: Stand in an upright, relaxed posture with your knees loosely bent. Stretch your arms overhead, first one and then the other. Feel your ribs and waist opening and releasing.

**2** Right: Now bring your arms out at shoulder level and swing round from the waist, first to one side and then the other, without changing your leg or arm position. Repeat both movements.

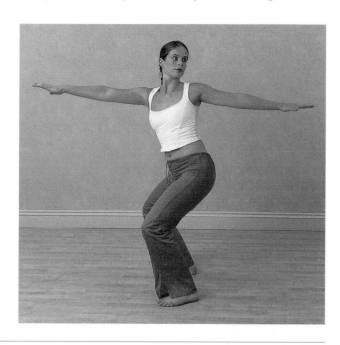

# Adapted easy triangle sequence

This sequence works out your abdominal muscles and increases flexibility in the lower spine. This can help to prevent backache and tone up your muscles. However, make sure that you proceed very gently.

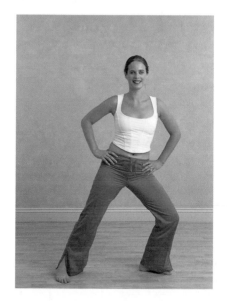

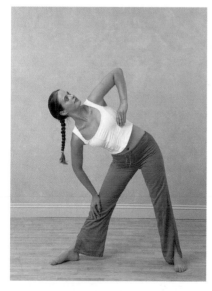

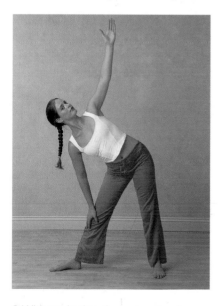

**1** Stand tall with feet wide and knees bent. Place your hands on your hips. Sway from side to side, tipping your pelvis up to the right as you sway to the right and up to the left as you sway to the left in a rhythmical movement. Keep your spine erect, coccyx tucked under and chest lifted. Repeat several times.

**2** Now bend to your right side without tipping forwards – keep your back straight and do not push yourself further than feels comfortable. Place your right hand along your leg and bring your left elbow back to open the left side of the waist and chest as you look up. Keep breathing rhythmically.

**3** Without losing the extension in your back, stretch your left arm up and back to open the left side of your body. Keep your abdomen relaxed and do not tense the right shoulder. Breathe deeply. Now come up slowly and repeat the bend on your left side. Do the exercise several times on both sides.

# Creating a balanced life

Being pregnant may mean that you have less energy than usual. It is very important to make time for relaxation and exercise, and this may mean that you have to make adjustments to your daily life.

Your list of priorities will probably run something like this:
- My health and my baby's health.
- My partner.
- My family and friends.
- Work commitments and any other must-do activities.
- Socializing.

Bear this list in mind if you are feeling overwhelmed. Decide what you are going to do – and remind yourself that you cannot do everything. Some things may need to be left undone, others may have to be delegated. Make the following your motto: prioritize, delegate, eliminate.

### YOUR QUALITY TIME

You are likely to feel tired when you are pregnant and coping with all the demands of everyday life can sometimes be difficult. Make sure that you prioritize time for yourself, or your own needs are likely to be eclipsed by home and work.

Think about what you would most enjoy, and what would help you to relax most. This could be singing, walking, going for acupuncture treatment, joining a pottery class, salsa, swimming or having a facial. Make sure that you incorporate regular 'me time' into your week so that you can do what gives you pleasure. In addition, make sure you spend at least half an hour, and preferably more, relaxing at home every day.

### SHORTCUTS AT HOME

Some things have to give when you are pregnant – and household chores are often a good place to compromise. Cut back so that you do the bare minimum. Ask your partner to do more, or consider hiring some extra help. Here are some good ways to reduce the time you spend.

### Shopping

Don't fritter away your time by shopping for food every day or two. Keep shopping down to the minimum – if possible, do one big shop per week. Ask your partner or a friend to come with you, or to do the shopping for you. Wherever possible, get your groceries delivered: investigate local vegetable-box schemes and shop via the Internet for non-perishable items that you don't need to select yourself. Buying teabags, toilet paper, washing

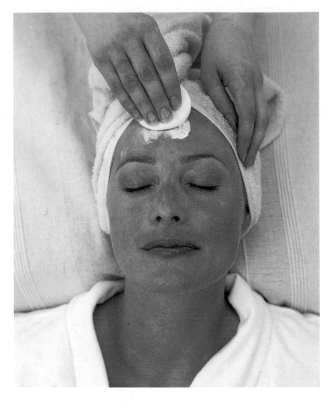

*View regular pampering as an important part of your pregnancy care. Relaxing moments and treats help to lift your spirits and raise your energy levels.*

powder, tins and other essential items in bulk can save you both time and money.

### Cooking

If you can get a good lunch during the working day, you may need only a healthy snack and lots of liquid in the evening. When cooking at home, concentrate on quick and easy, nutritious dishes rather than complex meals. Try the following:
- Home-made soups with wholemeal bread.
- Baked potato and cottage cheese.
- Fish risotto.
- Grilled bacon and tomatoes on wholemeal toast.
- Baked potato with baked beans and poached egg.
- Spaghetti with pancetta and tomatoes.
- Poached salmon with salad and new potatoes.
- Poached chicken with tomatoes and red peppers.
- Fish pie (if made in advance) and vegetables.
- Grilled trout with salad and new potatoes.
- Casseroles (beef, lamb, chicken) or other dishes that you can make ahead of time.

If you feel like a dessert, have something healthy such as:
- Fresh fruit and natural yogurt.
- Bananas and crème fraîche.
- Baked apples.

When cooking dishes such as casseroles or pasta sauces, make double the quantity and freeze the rest for another day. That way, you cook less often and will always have a stock of nourishing food in the house.

### Housework
- Wash clothes twice a week at most, and preferably only once.
- Change your bedlinen less often than usual. Once every 10–14 days is fine.
- Iron only what you really have to – don't worry about bedlinen, tea towels, hand towels, undersheets, duvet covers, underwear or T-shirts. If you take washing off the line or out of the dryer as soon as it is dry and fold it immediately, you should not have to iron.
- Remember that your home doesn't have to be pristine – a bit of dust won't harm you.

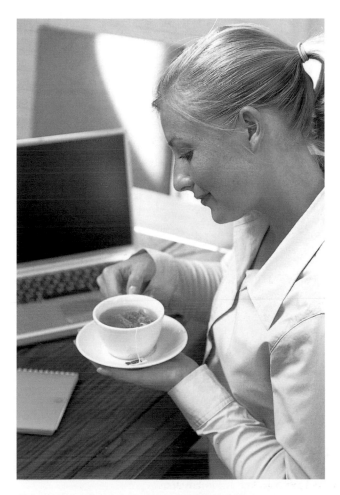

*Take regular time out when you are working – an afternoon break with a cup of herbal tea and a cereal bar can help to refresh you for the rest of the day.*

### GETTING ON TOP OF WORK
Many women find work a struggle, particularly in the early months of pregnancy when they may be feeling exhausted and nauseous. Here are some ways that can help to make it easier.
- Get to work a little early so that you have some quiet time to yourself to get your breath back from the journey, and have a nutritious drink (chamomile tea, for example, or fresh fruit juice).
- If you control your workload, tackle the most demanding jobs early in the day if possible. Remember the first rule of management: 'Don't touch any piece of paper more than once'. Deal with it, file it or bin it straight away. Treat emails in the same way.
- Do not stand for long periods at work – sit down whenever you can. If you work sitting down, stand up and stretch at regular intervals.
- Take at least 45 minutes for your lunch break. Make this a time to eat and rest rather than an opportunity to go shopping. If you feel very tired, see if you can find a place to take a nap.
- Be sure to get some fresh air at lunchtime – just walking once round the block will really help to refresh you – so that you don't start to feel sleepy halfway through the afternoon.
- Counter a mid-afternoon energy dip with a healthy cereal bar and a cup of herbal tea (keep your favourite herbal tea bags at work). If possible, use this time to do any easier jobs, such as making routine phone calls.
- Take your holiday as and when you should. Don't allow your holiday allocation to slip over from one year to the next.
- Take some of your holiday as single days – say, one day every couple of weeks. Use this time to rest, not to rush around trying to catch up at home.
- Take sick days if you need them. Don't struggle into work if you are feeling poorly. Consider telling your manager why you are taking time off.
- If feasible, work from home at least one day a week, in order to give you a break from travelling.
- When you get home from work, try not to jump straight into your next task. Instead, sit down for half an hour and rest, relax with the newspaper or a book, have a bath, or go for a walk.

> 66 Remind yourself that you cannot do everything. Some things may need to be left undone, others may have to be delegated. 99

# Routine antenatal care

By the eighth or ninth week of your pregnancy, you should have seen your family doctor and registered for antenatal care. If not, then make an appointment as soon as possible. Where you actually receive your antenatal care, and the type of care that you receive, is usually linked with where you ultimately want your baby to be delivered. The first consultation – commonly called the booking-in appointment – is usually held at the maternity unit of your local hospital, where you can discuss your future care. You will be referred here by your family doctor.

It is useful to have an idea of where you would like the baby to be born, and to have discussed this with your partner, before the first antenatal appointment. However, don't worry if you are not sure – there is plenty of time to make a decision and you can, of course, change your mind at a later date.

### HOSPITAL-BASED CARE

If you have chosen to have your baby in hospital, then you will probably see hospital staff two or three times during your whole pregnancy. Your family doctor or community midwife will undertake the rest of the care. You will probably be seen at the hospital for a booking-in appointment at around 10 to 12 weeks, then again at about 34 or 36 weeks and once more when your baby is finally due.

If you prefer all the antenatal visits to be carried out at the hospital where you will have your baby, your family doctor can arrange this for you.

### FAMILY DOCTOR OR COMMUNITY CARE

You may be able to have all your antenatal care in your family doctor's surgery or at the community midwives' office, particularly if you have decided to have your baby at home and so long as there are no problems with your pregnancy. You should discuss your preferences at the first booking appointment.

### DOMINO SCHEME

The word Domino stands for Domiciliary In/Out. This is a scheme in which a community midwife shares your antenatal care with the hospital and your family doctor, sometimes visiting you at home to do the routine antenatal checks. The midwife will look after you at home, take you into hospital, deliver your baby and then arrange for you to return home within 48 hours of the birth.

### MIDWIFE DELIVERY

You may choose to have a midwife be responsible for all your antenatal care and the delivery. In this case, you may not see a doctor during your pregnancy, except for the initial referral and unless the midwife becomes concerned about the pregnancy.

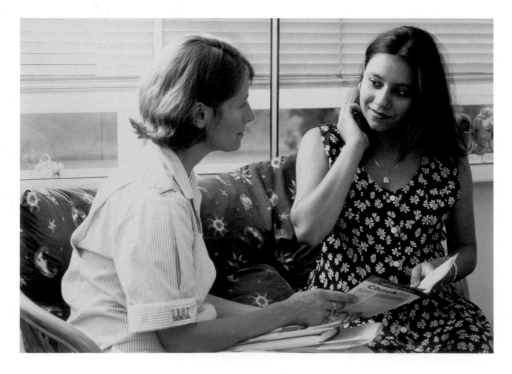

*Your midwife or doctor should be happy to discuss any fears or questions that you have about your pregnancy.*

## TESTS

By around 12 weeks, you will have an appointment at your antenatal clinic – probably the first of several. This first visit is intended to ascertain whether or not your pregnancy and delivery are likely to be normal. Routine checks will be done, including your weight, blood pressure, urine and blood. You may be offered an HIV test. The midwife will examine your abdomen to check the size of your uterus.

You can discuss screening procedures during this visit and are likely to be offered a routine ultrasound scan, usually done around weeks 10 to 12, to check the baby is developing normally. There are other diagnostic tests available, such as nuchal fold ultrasound, triple alphafetoprotein (AFP) and amniocentesis. You don't need to decide what tests, if any, you would like to go ahead with straight away: take time to consider the options.

## YOUR FIRST ULTRASOUND

You will be asked to drink a pint of water before your appointment so that you have a full bladder for the ultrasound. This causes the uterus to be pushed outwards so that it – and the baby – can be clearly seen.

You lie down for the scan with your abdomen bared. Your skin is covered with a gel, because soundwaves cannot travel through air. The sensor or probe has to make direct airtight contact with your skin. The probe is placed on your abdomen and you will see an almost incomprehensible picture on a screen next to you.

The operator will explain what you can see. You should be able to see the baby moving and you will see its heart beating from the seventh week and hear it from the tenth week. Because the baby is so small, it is not possible to see if it is a boy or girl at this stage.

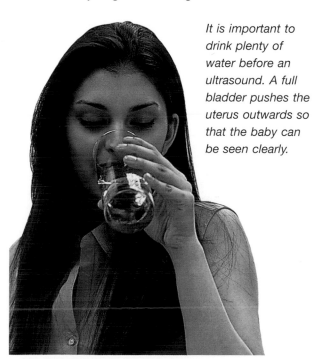

*It is important to drink plenty of water before an ultrasound. A full bladder pushes the uterus outwards so that the baby can be seen clearly.*

## WHO'S WHO IN THE ANTENATAL TEAM

These are the people who may be involved in your pregnancy care:

- **Consultant obstetrician:** senior hospital specialist in charge of maternity care.

- **Consultant pediatrician:** senior hospital specialist in charge of newborn babies and children.

- **Registrar:** senior doctor who is junior to the consultant and resident in the hospital.

- **Senior house officer:** junior hospital doctor undertaking next level of training and able to call upon the registrar for advice if necessary.

- **Midwife:** nurse specializing in the management of normal pregnancy and labour.

- **Family doctor:** many family doctors undertake much of the antenatal work but few supervise delivery.

- **Health visitor:** about ten days after midwife care finishes, the health visitor takes over. She will advise on the care of your baby and help you deal with any problems.

- **Anaesthetist:** doctor specially trained in giving general and local anaesthesia, including epidurals.

- **Radiologist:** doctor who interprets pictures from imaging techniques, such as X-rays and ultrasounds.

- **Radiographer:** health professional, not a doctor, who performs imaging techniques.

- **Physiotherapist:** health professional who teaches antenatal care and exercises, helps to combat the pain of labour and is skilled in teaching muscle-strengthening exercises and dealing with other ligament and joint problems that occur during or after pregnancy.

- **Social worker:** assists with social problems that may occur during or after pregnancy. Social workers have special counselling skills for women who have emotional or social problems and bridge the gap between the family doctor and the health visitor.

- **Medical students:** may observe antenatal care, labour and delivery as part of their training. Students are required to undertake a certain number of normal deliveries under supervision and to learn certain procedures such as repairing an episiotomy. You have the right to ask for students not to be present.

# Tests and specialist care

It is natural to worry about whether your baby is developing normally, but remind yourself that around 97 per cent of pregnancies end in the safe delivery of a healthy baby – and that your antenatal team is there to ensure that any problems are picked up quickly. As well as routine antenatal care, you will be offered diagnostic tests, used to identify serious problems with the baby.

## SPECIALIST TESTS
Many women find it reassuring to have diagnostic tests done, but some do not. You are under no obligation to have any of the tests you are offered: you and your partner have the right to decide what is best for you. It is important to remember that no test is 100 per cent accurate, and tests cannot detect all abnormalities.

### Chorionic villus sampling
This test is usually carried out at nine to ten weeks (or at any rate not after week 13) and can be used to diagnose Down's syndrome. It can also detect the same chromosome abnormalities as amniocentesis and other genetic disorders such as sickle-cell anaemia and thalassaemia. It is also possible to detect the sex of the

> **"** Around 97 per cent of pregnancies end in the safe delivery of a healthy baby. **"**

fetus and this may be of value if there is a known sex-linked condition in the family.

A narrow plastic tube is passed into the uterus through the cervix and some cells from the developing placenta are drawn off. Some doctors may insert a needle through the abdominal wall rather like amniocentesis, using ultrasound to guide them. The results should be known after ten days. The risk of miscarriage after the test is one in 100, which is higher than with amniocentesis.

### Nuchal fold ultrasound
The nuchal fold ultrasound is also known as the nuchal fold or the translucency scan. It is done at about 11–14 weeks, and it is used to predict Down's syndrome cases. The procedure is the same as that for a routine ultrasound, but the operator concentrates on getting a good image of the fetus's neck on the screen and then measures a layer of fluid at the back of the neck. The thicker this layer is, the greater the chance the baby will have Down's syndrome. The chance or risk is expressed as a probability such as a one in 10,000 chance or a one in 100 chance. Depending on the risk identified, you may be advised to have further tests such as amniocentesis.

### Doppler ultrasound
This ultrasound is an advanced form of ultrasound imaging and is available only in some specialist hospitals. It can be used to diagnose more accurately the well-being of the baby if previous tests have shown that it is not growing sufficiently well.

The Doppler scanner can identify the veins and arteries through which blood flows and can detect the speed at which the blood is travelling. As this indicates how much oxygen the baby is receiving, it also predicts if a placenta is not functioning well. Colour Doppler is a more sophisticated technique than standard Doppler, and its benefits are still being evaluated.

### Later tests
Amniocentesis or the alphafetoprotein test may also be offered as part of your antenatal care. These tests are carried out in the second trimester – see pages 68–71.

---

**WHAT IS DOWN'S SYNDROME?**
Normal babies have 23 pairs of chromosomes: 46 in total. In Down's syndrome, there is an extra chromosome – usually in the 21st pair. This causes various physical and mental abnormalities.

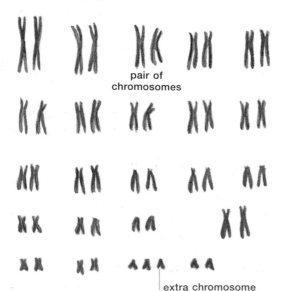

pair of chromosomes

extra chromosome

---

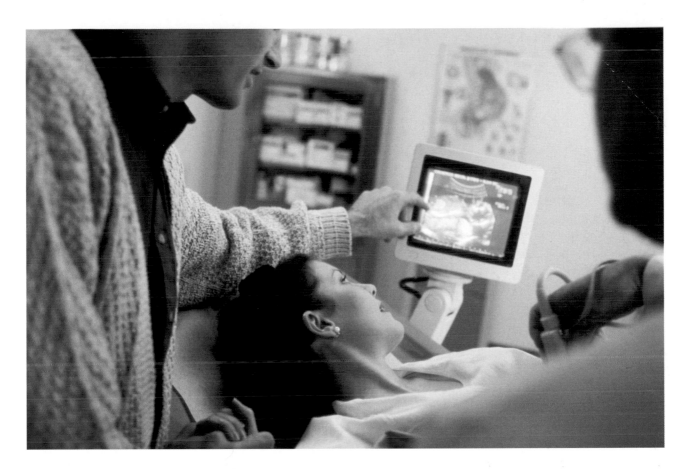

## RISK FACTORS

Some women have a higher risk of carrying a baby with abnormalities than others. Doctors have identified certain risk factors, including the mother's age, her or her partner's medical history and the outcome of previous pregnancies. These factors do not mean that you will develop problems in this pregnancy, only that you have a statistically higher risk of doing so than women who are not affected by the same risk factors. Because of this, you may be monitored more closely by the medical team.

## TWINS AND MULTIPLE PREGNANCIES

If you are expecting twins or more, you will be more closely monitored throughout your pregnancy. You will probably need more assistance during and after the delivery, so a home birth may not be advisable. Fatigue and nausea may be increased throughout the pregnancy. Twin or multiple pregnancies are usually shorter than the norm: about 37 weeks rather than 40.

## INHERITED DISEASES

You should tell the doctor at your first antenatal check if any of the following or any inherited diseases are known in your family or in your partner's family:

- Single gene defects such as Huntington's chorea/disease, cystic fibrosis and sickle-cell anaemia.
- Disorders linked to damage on the X-chromosome such as haemophilia and muscular dystrophy.

*During an ultrasound, the operator will explain what you can see on the screen. You will be able to ask any questions that you have and discuss the findings.*

- Chromosomal defects such as Down's syndrome.
- Neural tube defects, which include anencephaly and spina bifida.

## GENETIC COUNSELLING

You may be offered this to assess the likelihood of certain problems in your pregnancy. It is most often offered to:

- Women over the age of 35, because there is an greater risk of the baby being affected by Down's.
- Parents of a child with a genetic abnormality, a neural tube defect or other form of physical impairment.
- Women who have a tendency to miscarry.
- Couples with known chromosome abnormalities.
- Women who may be carriers of X-linked disorders (such as haemophilia).
- Couples whose family members have a high incidence of a certain disease.
- Couples whose ethnic or racial backgrounds increase the likelihood of a particular problem such as sickle-cell anaemia, thalassaemia or Tay-Sachs disease.

If you believe you need genetic counselling but you have not been offered it, discuss the reasons with your family doctor or consultant.

# Possible problems

A large number of pregnancies proceed with no serious difficulties, but things can go wrong. Two of the main problems are ectopic pregnancies and miscarriage.

### ECTOPIC PREGNANCY

An ectopic pregnancy is one that starts to develop in one of the Fallopian tubes or, more rarely, in another site in the abdominal cavity rather than in the uterus. It can cause permanent damage to the tube, leading to infertility. Doctors do not know why an ectopic pregnancy occurs. However, it is more common if the Fallopian tube has already been damaged by infection, surgery or by a previous ectopic pregnancy.

An ectopic pregnancy can be extremely serious, even life-threatening, and so the woman must get immediate medical treatment. The symptoms can include intense pain in the abdominal area and vaginal bleeding. Ectopic pregnancies are sometimes initially diagnosed as appendicitis or miscarriage.

An ectopic pregnancy cannot develop normally. Once an ectopic pregnancy is confirmed, surgery is needed to remove it. Sometimes, part of the Fallopian tube and part

> **" At these difficult times it is essential that partners are totally supportive of each other "**

of the ovary may have to be removed as well, although doctors will avoid this whenever possible. Women who have suffered one ectopic pregnancy are at a higher risk of experiencing another one. However, many women who have had an ectopic pregnancy go on to have a perfectly healthy pregnancy.

### MISCARRIAGE

A high proportion of miscarriages occur within the first two months of pregnancy, often before the woman knows that she is pregnant. The loss of a baby through early miscarriage is much more common than many people believe (it may also account for many cases of what is thought to be delayed conception). Some experts believe that as many as over a half of all early pregnancies could be ending in miscarriage.

The warning signs for an impending miscarriage are similar to the symptoms of a menstrual period and include vaginal bleeding, abdominal cramps and backache. Excessive vomiting can also be a symptom. Once a miscarriage starts, there is little that can be done to halt it. However, it is important that you seek medical advice immediately because there is a risk of infection and other complications.

### INVESTIGATING MISCARRIAGE

Having a miscarriage can be a very traumatic experience. For some women it is just as distressing as a bereavement, even when it occurs in the early stages of pregnancy. It may be of some comfort to know that miscarriage, particularly in the early months, is very common. It does not mean that there is anything inherently wrong with you, or that you are likely to miscarry next time you become pregnant. The vast majority of women go on to have successful pregnancies after experiencing a miscarriage. For this reason, having one or even two early miscarriages is not usually seen as a reason for medical investigation.

Tests are usually done if a woman experiences repeated miscarriages: this is defined as three or more successive miscarriages with no successful pregnancy occurring in between. After suffering three miscarriages,

---

### ECTOPIC PREGNANCY

Sometimes a pregnancy can start to develop in the Fallopian tubes rather than in the uterus. An ectopic pregnancy is normally accompanied by severe abdominal pain, and the woman will need emergency treatment to remove the pregnancy.

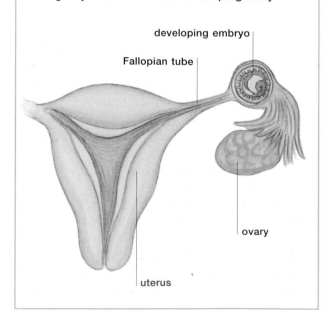

developing embryo

Fallopian tube

ovary

uterus

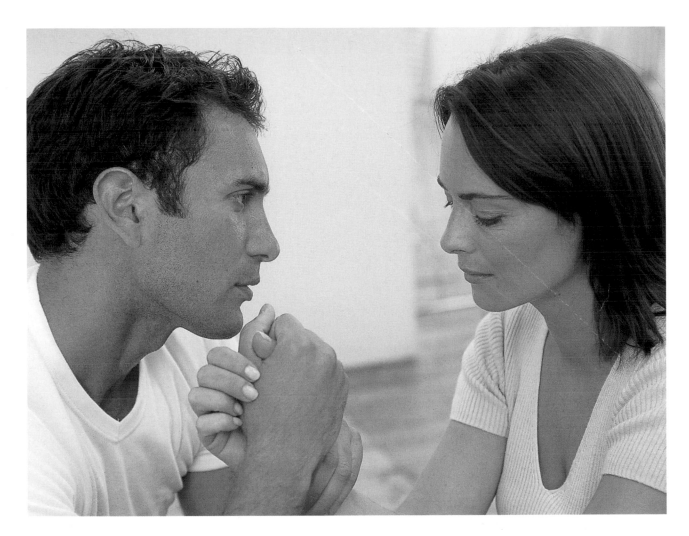

you should seek specialist help and advice. A late miscarriage – one that occurs after 14 weeks – should also be investigated.

Your family doctor will be able to refer you to a consultant gynaecologist if you have had recurrent miscarriages. In some cases, couples may then be referred to a genetic counsellor for further investigation. Genetic counselling may help to determine the level of risk to future pregnancies, and also to discuss the best way forwards.

## WHY MISCARRIAGE HAPPENS

Doctors still do not know why so many pregnancies end unsuccessfully, and determining the cause of a miscarriage can be extremely difficult – or even impossible. Some of the known causes of early miscarriage include:
- A major abnormality in the baby. About three in every five early miscarriages are thought to be connected to fetal abnormality.
- The mother contracting rubella, listeriosis or chlamydia during the pregnancy.
- The failure of the fertilized egg to implant successfully in the lining of the uterus.

*It can be very distressing for both parents-to-be when there are any problems with the smooth progression of a pregnancy. At these difficult times it is essential that partners are totally supportive of each other.*

- The mother having a low level of progesterone, which is needed to sustain the pregnancy.

Later miscarriage (after 14 weeks) can be the result of:
- An abnormality in the uterus, such as a large fibroid (fibroids are bundles of muscle fibres that have developed in the muscular wall of the uterus).
- A weak (incompetent) cervix. This is a condition in which the cervix dilates instead of remaining tightly closed during pregnancy.
- Certain antenatal tests; amniocentesis, for example, carries a 1 in 200 risk of miscarriage.
- The mother having diabetes, epilepsy, asthma, kidney disease or high blood pressure.

Miscarriages are more common in very young women or women over 35. Many people think that minor injuries or distress can cause a miscarriage, but there is no medical evidence to support this.

# Checklist of common problems

The first trimester brings its own distinct symptoms. Many first-trimester complaints can be eased by complementary therapies, but always seek advice from a qualified therapist and check any therapies and remedies with your midwife or doctor.

If a complaint persists or troubles you, or you are not sure what it is, consult your family doctor. In any case, mention any problem at your next antenatal check. Do not take any over-the-counter drugs (or prescription drugs left over from pre-pregnancy) unless you have checked that they are safe in pregnancy with the pharmacist, your doctor or a consultant.

**Anxiety**  There are many things that women worry about while pregnant, and anxiety is especially common during the early stages of pregnancy because the whole experience is new and unfamiliar and also because miscarriage is most common during the first trimester. Discuss particular worries or persistent anxiety with your doctor or midwife. You will also find that breathing exercises and meditation will lower general anxiety levels very effectively.

**Bleeding**  Bleeding or spotting is not uncommon during the first three months. The cause may never be found or it may spring from a variety of causes, such as a minor infection. However, there may be more potentially dangerous reasons, so always get any bleeding or spotting checked out.

**Breast soreness**  One of the classic early signs of pregnancy, sore, sensitive or unusually tender breasts can be relieved greatly by a professionally fitted maternity bra. You will find that this symptom usually eases after the first trimester.

**Fainting**  You may feel slight faintness alongside morning sickness and a general feeling of being under par. However, if faintness is persistent or regular, or you actually faint or feel like you are going to, then you should drink plenty of water and consult your family doctor without delay.

**Fatigue**  Tiredness is the frequent complaint of many pregnant women, particularly during the first trimester, when hormonal changes put the woman's body under unfamiliar strains. The simple answer is to make sure that you go to bed earlier and take naps whenever you

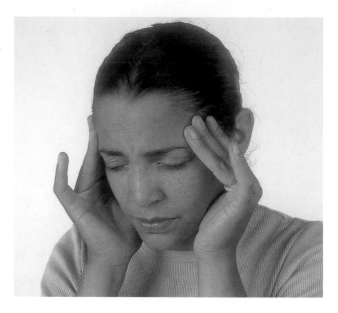

*Headaches are a regular occurrence for many pregnant women, and may accompany the general feelings of being unwell that often occur in the first trimester. Acupressure can be especially helpful in esing symptoms, but always seek out professional advice about using this.*

can. However, fatigue can be a symptom of anaemia, so extreme tiredness should be always be checked out properly by a doctor.

**Headache**  Troublesome headaches are another symptom that can accompany general under-par feelings in early pregnancy, as hormonal changes make themselves felt. If headaches persist for more than two days, you must consult your family doctor without delay.

Acupuncture can be a useful therapeutic tool in relieving headaches. Massage can prove very effective, because it relieves the muscle tension that causes so many headaches and also improves blood circulation. Chamomile tea soothes headache symptoms, as can lavender oil – just three or four drops on a compress, applied to the temples. Good homeopathic remedies to try include calc carb, arsen alb, and nux vomica.

**Insomnia**  Many women have problems sleeping during pregnancy – at first because of bodily changes and perhaps early anxiety, and then later because the increasing bulk of your growing baby can make it difficult to find a comfortable position. Perhaps the most important strategy here is to establish a regular night-time routine – for example, have a warm bath and a milky drink at night and go to bed at the same time. Do not eat late at night and avoid salty, sugary, fatty and spicy foods. Do not drink tea or coffee at night, as the caffeine is over-stimulating; chamomile tea is a very soothing night-time drink. Getting into these good habits as early as possible during pregnancy will mean that you don't suddenly have to impose them later on.

Complementary therapies have much to offer where insomnia is concerned. Ask your partner to give you a gentle massage in the evening. Walk or swim regularly, early in the morning or during the day, perhaps at lunchtime. A medical herbalist, homeopath or acupuncturist may also be able to help.

**Morning sickness** This is the main symptom associated with the first trimester and includes general feelings of nausea and actual vomiting. Despite its name, this sickness is not confined to mornings – some women feel nauseous only in the evening, some only in the morning and some at intervals all through the day.

The precise cause of morning sickness is unknown, but is assumed to relate to hormonal changes. Start the day with dry toast and a cup of tea. Eat light meals and take small, frequent drinks. Avoid fats and fatty and spicy foods. Reiki may help, and you might also like to consult a medical herbalist or a homeopath – good homeopathic remedies include ipecac, nux vomica and pulsatilla. (See also pages 16–17.)

**Stretchmarks** Marks caused by stretching of the skin as your baby grows are common during pregnancy, and may persist afterwards. Get into the habit of moisturizing this area as early on as possible, so that, when the skin starts to be stretched, it is supple and marking is minimal. To do this, massage the abdomen, thighs and buttocks regularly (and gently) with vitamin E oil.

**Urinary infection** This is common in pregnancy, but should always be treated without delay. Signs include the need to race to the lavatory, burning or stinging upon urination, a need to pass urine frequently, difficulty in passing urine or passing urine flecked with blood. See your doctor straight away if you have any of these symptoms or suspect the possibility of infection.

In order to allay infection, make sure that you always drink plenty of water. Cranberry juice is very effective at keeping the urinary tract healthy and able to stave off potential problems.

**Urination, frequent** This is something most women have to put up with in pregnancy and especially during the first trimester. It is typically caused by hormone changes and the growing uterus pushing on the bladder

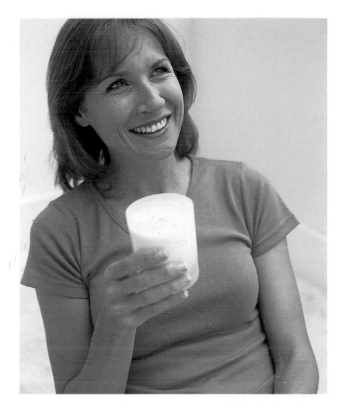

*Milky drinks taken before bedtime may help to ease the insomnia that so often accompanies early pregnancy.*

and decreasing its size. Do not drink less as this can lead to an infected urinary tract. In fact, the frequent urination may actually be caused by a urinary infection – tell your doctor if you have any signs of this (see above).

**Vaginal discharge** Consult your family doctor straight away if you notice unusual or heavy discharge.

This long list may make it seem as though pregnancy is fraught with problems. However, the great majority of women do not experience any serious difficulties. Many symptoms, including nausea, will not last long. They can be uncomfortable but most have no serious effects.

**SEEKING ADVICE**
If you are worried by any symptom, do not hesitate to call or visit your doctor.
See your doctor straight away if you have:
- A high temperature (38.5°C/101°F or above).
- Swelling of the hands and ankles.
Seek emergency assistance if you have:
- Vaginal bleeding other than spotting.
- Severe abdominal pain.
- Excessive vomiting.
- Sudden swelling of the hands and ankles or blurred vision with a severe headache.

# Common Qs and As

**Q: My partner and I are expecting our first baby in about six months' time, but he does not seem as excited as I am. Should I be worried?**

A: Many men do not fully appreciate the wonder of new life until the baby is actually born and named: in other words when the baby has a tangible identity. This probably sounds awful to the newly pregnant woman, but don't despair. Once the baby is born, the man is usually fantastically proud, wanting to show off his little girl or little boy to everyone.

**Q: My mother and my mother-in-law keep dropping broad hints about our starting a family – and we ourselves have wanted this for a long time. Now I am pregnant, but I am loath to tell anyone until I am absolutely sure everything is all right. Both of us are finding the pressure hard to take. What should we do?**

A: Carry on fending off their enquiries as best you can. They will understand once you get to the 12th week and tell them the happy news. A word of warning, though: don't let them take over your pregnancy with lots of well-meaning advice. Tell them you that want to do things your own way and remind them that you are receiving good antenatal care. When the baby comes along, remind yourself that it is your child, not theirs, and set boundaries if you have to. Go with your own instincts about what to do – or seek professional advice.

**Q: We had not intended to start a family quite so soon and my pregnancy has taken us both by surprise. Now the weeks seem to be whizzing by and I feel as if I cannot quite catch up. What can I do?**

A: How lovely not to have to plan when to start your family. Don't worry, you and your partner will soon be rejoicing in your good fortune. In the meantime, make a list of all the things that you think you would like to do before the baby comes. Consider whether all these tasks are essential – if not, eliminate them. Work out how you will achieve these, month by month, making allowances for the fact that you will be feeling tired, especially in the latter months of pregnancy. Consider what you can delegate to others, and what you want to do yourself.

**Q: I am not sure if I want all the tests to do with antenatal care but I don't know what to say to the doctor.**

A: One of the benefits of having the tests is to receive confirmation that there is nothing wrong with the baby. Another benefit is that some problems can be treated in the uterus. Alternatively, hospital staff may arrange to have relevant specialists on hand at the delivery if they know of a potential problem. They will also arrange for the baby's well-being to be monitored through the hours of labour and delivery, and, if necessary, they will perform a Caesarean.

You are not obliged to have any test – and some women feel strongly that they do not want to do so. The best thing to do is to talk over your feelings with your midwife or family doctor so that he or she understands your perspective and can advise you accordingly. You can take your partner or a good friend to the appointment if you feel you need extra support. It can also be helpful to contact natural childbirth organizations for a different point of view.

Q: We are expecting twins and don't know how to tell our two-year-old the news. We are also worried how he will react when the twins arrive, since he will inevitably receive less attention in the future than he has been used to. What do you advise?

A: Children can become very excited about the birth of a brother or sister, even if they subsequently feel rather jealous of them. It's a good idea to tell children about a pregnancy when it is advanced enough to be visible. Show him your bump and let him touch it. Explain that there is a baby inside – he might like to try to talk to it. Show him any scan pictures you have as well. As your pregnancy progresses, your son will enjoy feeling the baby kick.

The fact that you have anticipated problems after the birth is half the battle. Your little boy may feel somewhat eclipsed because twins do demand a lot of attention, and they usually attract wonder and admiration from friends and family.

You need to keep in mind your little boy's need to be admired himself, and express daily your love for him. Perhaps you could arrange for someone else to look after the twins for a short period each day so that you can concentrate on your little boy.

Two is not an easy age in any case, when your little boy will, quite naturally, start to express his independence. Signs of temper and disobedience are all part of this and will not necessarily be related to the birth of the twins. Chat to your health visitor about this when the time comes so that she can give you useful tips for your individual situation.

Q: I have a hugely demanding job and cannot imagine how I can cope with pregnancy and then look after a small baby while I continue to work.

A: First, you will be on maternity leave – perhaps for as long as six months or a year. Second, someone else will be doing your job while you are away. Third, you will find that the pregnancy hormones will have the effect of slowing you down. While it may seem unthinkable at the moment, you will find ways of reducing the work demands made upon you as time goes on.

Ultimately, you will be compelled to make some difficult choices. Will you give up your job and stay at home? Could you job-share? Would working part-time be an option? Could you return to work full-time six weeks or so after the baby's birth and have a childminder or a nanny? Could you get help in the home to help you to cope?

You will not know what is really right for you until after the delivery of the baby. For the time being, concentrate on your work and your pregnancy, and deal with any problems only when and if they arise.

Q: I am self-employed and will need to return to work quite quickly after the birth. How can I keep my clients happy in the last month of my pregnancy and in those first few weeks?

A: You will need to cut down the hours that you work for a few weeks before the delivery, and you will not be able to return for a few weeks afterwards. Tell your clients your situation when you are about six months pregnant, so that you can prepare them for your absence. It may be worth employing someone to cover for you, or to take over essential administration. Avoid becoming overtired; stick to early nights and catnap in the afternoon if you can.

# CHAPTER TWO
# The second trimester

" Many women find that they are glowing with good health and vitality. "

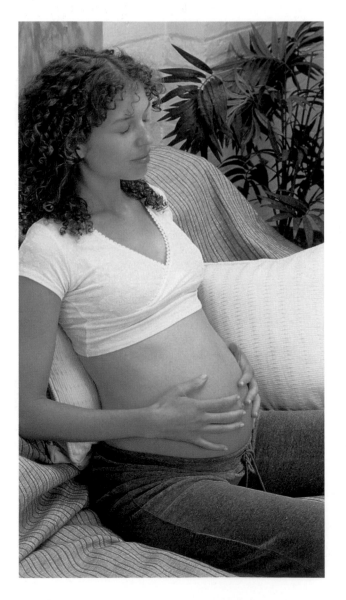

The second three months are often the best and the happiest stage of a woman's pregnancy. You are now past the early weeks in which the chance of miscarriage is high, and the 12-week scan is already behind you. This is the best stage at which to enjoy your pregnancy and start making plans for the birth.

By this time, most women are no longer suffering from sickness and the overwhelming fatigue brought on by the hormonal changes of the first few weeks. Better still, many women find that they are glowing with good health and vitality. You will most likely experience a growing sensation of well-being during the second trimester, and you may well look as good as you feel. Your eyes may shine, your hair may be thick and lustrous, and your skin may be clear, smooth and luminous.

This is an exciting period, too. You and your partner can see your body changing from week to week, and with each week passing you are better able to visualize your growing baby. You are likely to

*As the second trimester progresses, you can watch your baby growing week by week. The extra weight may cause tiredness, so rest whenever you can.*

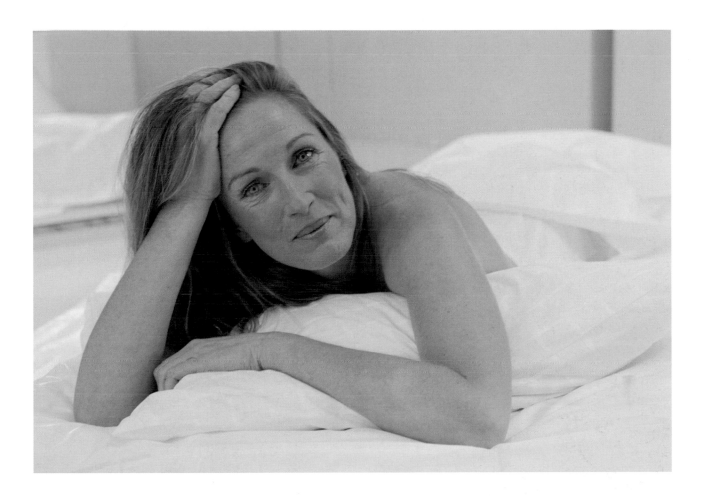

be very physically aware of your pregnancy, but as yet the baby is not big enough to slow you down too much and prevent you from doing the things that you want to do. Enjoy it.

Continue to look after yourself as well as possible. Be aware that the steadily increasing size of the baby inside you is starting to place pressure on your spine. This may lead to backache and extreme tiredness if you don't take preventative steps. Check your posture at all times, standing tall and sitting with your back firmly upright and supported. Yoga will help to strengthen your back at this stage, and this is also valuable preparation for labour. Similarly, Alexander technique classes can provide many tips for relaxed but upright postures and movement.

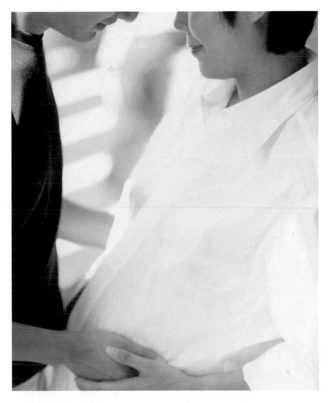

*Top: For many women, the second trimester brings a wonderful sense of well-being, with morning sickness a thing of the past and a new lustre to skin and hair.*

*This is the time to enjoy your pregnancy to the full. Share the excitement and sensations of each new development with those closest to you.*

# Growth from twelve weeks

By the end of the third month of pregnancy (12 or 13 weeks), your baby has become a recognizable human being. All the body's structures and organs have formed. Your baby's arms and legs, fingers and toes have all developed, although they are still very small.

The baby's sexual characteristics are developing at this time. The boy's penis is emerging, while a girl's cervix, vagina, uterus and ovaries will already have formed. If the baby is a girl, she will at the moment have in her ovaries about 4–5 million eggs, a number that drops to 2–3 million by the time she is born.

The baby's heartbeat is stronger; it is not yet audible with a stethoscope, but it can be heard with a hand-held electronic device. The placenta has started to function, giving your baby the nourishment he or she needs. Your baby will start to practise breathing movements for the first time between weeks 12 and 16.

During the second trimester of your pregnancy, your baby will be developing at an astonishing rate. He or she will increase in weight from 10g to over 600g (¼oz to 1lb 5oz). This growth will be reflected in your growing size and in your continued need for rest.

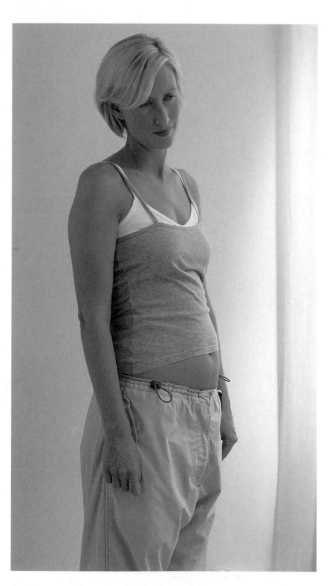

*At the start of the second trimester – which spans weeks 13 or 14 to around week 26 – the baby is still tiny and so you probably won't have a bump.*

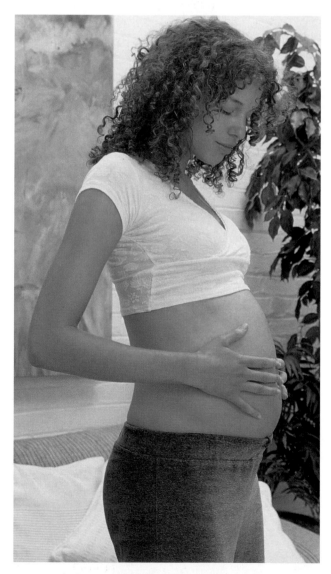

*As your pregnancy develops, you will see your belly growing more noticeable. By the end of this second term, you will be quite obviously pregnant.*

At week 12, your baby is about 60mm (2½in) long, measured from the crown of the head to the rump. He or she weighs about 9–13g (¼–½oz). He or she will have doubled in size in the last three weeks.

By now your baby is able to move his or her jaw and yawn. He or she can also suck and swallow – vital preparation for the life ahead. It is also around this time that the fingernails and toenails start to develop.

## Week 13

The length of your baby, measured from crown to rump, will be about 65–80mm (2½–3¼in). If you include the legs as well, his or her length will be 100mm (4in). He or she will weigh about 14–20g (½–¾oz). The eyelids meet and fuse together. They will not now open again for several weeks. An ultrasound taken at this time may show that your baby now puts a thumb in his or her mouth. The baby's skin is transparent and rosy red in colour, because you can see the blood vessels beneath the skin. The skeleton is becoming stronger, hardening as cartilage gradually develops into bone.

## Week 14

The baby now measures about 80–115mm (3¼–4¼in), crown to rump and weighs about 25g (1oz). The face is well developed with all the facial features recognizable. The cheeks and bridge of the nose appear, the ears move to a higher position on the head, and the eyes come closer together. As the baby develops more muscle tissue, he or she starts twisting and kicking and waving the arms within the amniotic sac. You are unlikely to feel your baby's movements because he or she still has plenty of space in which to splash around. A baby responds to gentle touch at this stage, and also moves away from threatening stimuli. During amniocentesis, babies have been seen to move away from the needle.

## Week 15

Your baby is now a recognizable human being, but he or she is not yet capable of independent life. The baby weighs about 80g (2¾oz) and is 10cm (4in) long. His or her fingernails are developing.

### GOING PUBLIC

Your pregnancy is bound to become obvious during the second trimester, not least because your bump is increasingly difficult to hide. You are past the most dangerous time for miscarriage, and will very probably have had the 12-week scan. This should give you the reassurance that your baby is growing normally. Now is the time to share your good news with family and friends, and to start making plans for the future.

## EARLY SECOND TRIMESTER

The baby's rapid development is sustained by a constant supply of nutrients, drawn from the mother's blood supply via the umbilical cord, and a network of blood vessels in the placenta.

### WEEK 14

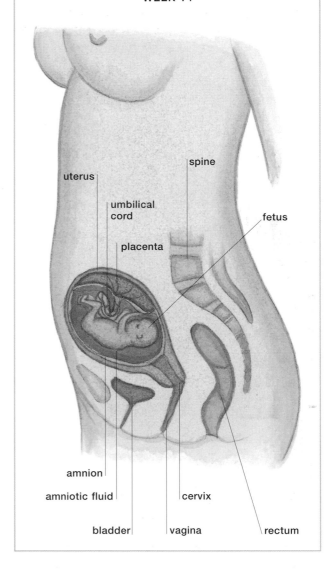

spine
uterus
umbilical cord
fetus
placenta
amnion
amniotic fluid
cervix
bladder
vagina
rectum

## Week 16

Your baby is now growing and gaining weight very quickly, He or she has grown to about 16cm (6in) in length and weighs about 110g (3¾oz). The baby is now moving around a great deal, although you are still unable to feel these movements. The baby's head is able to turn, the mouth open and the chest and stomach move up and down as if he or she were breathing deeply. The baby can also yawn and stretch, and even frown.

There is a growth of fine hair, known as lanugo, all over the baby's body. The head still looks very large compared with the rest of the body. The placenta is now completely developed. The baby's tiny toenails are forming.

### Week 17

A baby now weighs about 150g (5oz), and the reproductive organs are fully formed. The baby passes water containing waste products every 40–45 minutes. Much of this waste passes through the placenta and into your own circulation. You then excrete it through your urine and sweat.

### Weeks 18–19

By now your baby weighs about 200g (11oz). Between now and the 20th week, you may become aware of the baby's movements, which will feel like soft ripples. The arms and legs are well formed, and he or she does a lot of kicking, bumping, twisting and turning within the amniotic sac. The baby is able to move quite freely within the sac, and is lying in salt water, which gives extra buoyancy. The wall of the uterus is springy, so the baby can push against it with the feet, hands or head, then bounce off it.

Many babies are especially energetic in the evening when their mothers are more relaxed. You are most likely to feel the first signs of life – a little kick – at this time.

One of the most exciting thoughts of all is the fact that your baby is now able to make simple facial expressions, such as pleasure and distaste. His or her tastebuds are starting to form.

### Weeks 20–23

The baby now measures 25cm (10in) in length, and he or she weighs between 260g and 280g (9–10oz). His or her head is still large in proportion to the rest of the body: this signifies the brain's spectacular importance in all aspects of the baby's development. The teeth are beginning to form in the jawbone, and the hair is starting to grow.

By this stage, your baby will be completely covered in an oily layer known as vernix. The vernix comprises fatty

---

### CONTINUING DEVELOPMENT

By the end of the second trimester, the baby is well developed, with hair, fingernails and eyelashes all in place. His or her movements have become increasingly energetic. The baby's eyes will open for short periods in the next month. He or she will be able to see light, and will be aware of different sounds.

WEEK 20

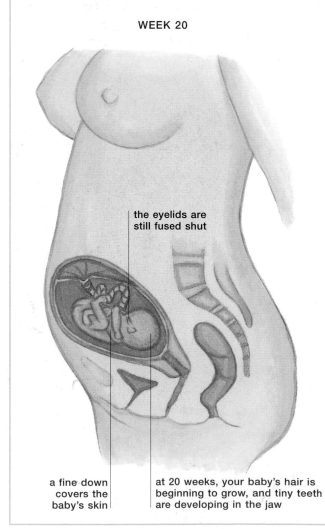

the eyelids are still fused shut

a fine down covers the baby's skin

at 20 weeks, your baby's hair is beginning to grow, and tiny teeth are developing in the jaw

WEEK 24

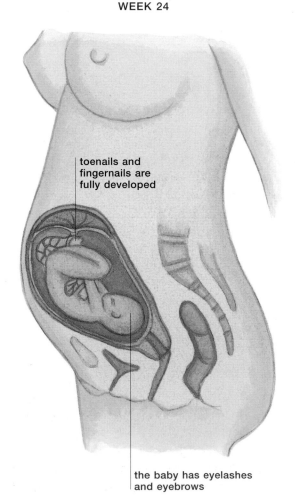

toenails and fingernails are fully developed

the baby has eyelashes and eyebrows

---

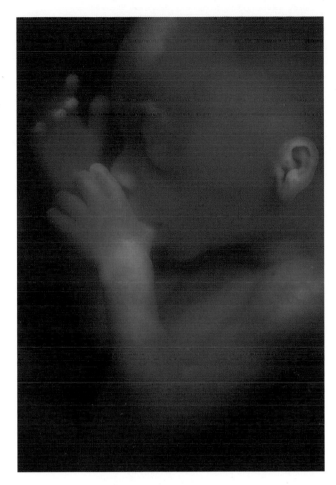

*This detailed scan shows the baby's hands up by her face. She may be sucking her thumb at this stage in an instinctive action that helps prepare for feeding later on.*

material and dead skin cells. This acts as a protective coating (in a sense, waterproofing the skin against the amniotic fluid). It remains present until the birth, when it helps to protect the baby during his or her passage down the birth canal and delivery into the outside world.

You may now be very conscious of your baby's movements, which feel like fluttering. At around this 20-week point, the key ultrasound scan – the mid-pregnancy one – is done. Most hospitals recommend this so that they can be well prepared for any problems that may arise at delivery time.

### Week 24

The baby is well developed in most respects by now, but his or her lungs are not capable of functioning fully. A baby born at this stage stands a reasonable chance of survival, but would need to remain in an intensive baby care unit and be given assistance with breathing.

The baby is getting longer and is still quite thin. Creases are visible on the palms and fingertips, and the skin is red and wrinkled. The fingernails have completely formed by now.

**❝** If your baby was to be born at 24 weeks, he or she would stand a reasonable chance of survival. **❞**

The baby may be sucking his or her thumb and may be hiccuping a lot. He or she is learning to co-ordinate sucking and swallowing in preparation for feeding after delivery. The organs of balance inside the ears have developed and are the same size as an adult's. The baby will be able to hear sounds from within and outside your body from about week 21, although it is very unlikely that he or she will be able to make sense of those sounds yet.

The baby's eyes begin to open occasionally but they do not remain open until about week 27. He or she now has delicate eyelashes and eyebrows, and can perceive light through the abdominal wall. The baby is now about 33cm (13in) in length. He or she has been gaining in weight rapidly in the last few weeks. Now that you are six months' pregnant, your baby will weigh approximately 570g–630g (1lb 3oz–1lb 6oz).

*Once the baby's weight starts to make itself felt, it can be all too tempting to slump, causing painful back problems. Always try to sit with your spine upright and your back properly supported.*

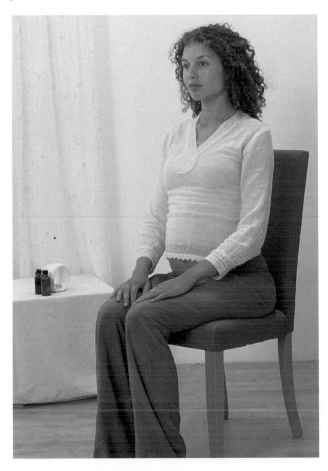

# How your body is changing

In the early weeks of the second trimester, you will feel very aware of your pregnancy. It will become obvious to other people at this stage, but you can still disguise the small bump by wearing loose clothing if you wish. You may still be suffering with morning sickness but this will almost certainly wear off very soon.

Your body will undergo many complex changes during the second trimester. Some of the changes that started in the first three months of your pregnancy will also become much more noticeable in the next few weeks.

At the beginning of this trimester, your uterus is the size of a large grapefruit; the top of the uterus will be swelling out just above your navel by the time you reach the third trimester. Food takes longer to digest now – about twice as long as before you were pregnant – so you may feel congested or bloated.

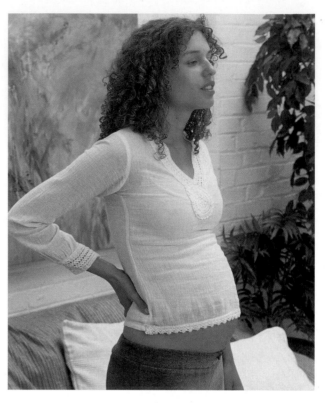

*Backache is common during pregnancy, so make sure that your back is always well supported.*

### STANDING TALL
You can alleviate backache to some extent by maintaining good posture. Keep your shoulders back but relaxed. Avoid jutting your head forwards; keep it back and tuck your jaw into your chin.

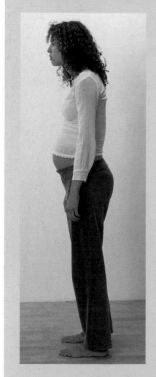

*This posture increases pressure on the spine.*

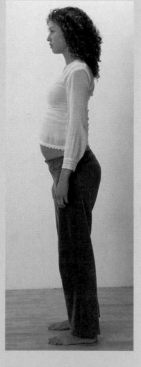

*Standing tall helps your back muscles.*

### COMMON SIGNS AND SOLUTIONS
Your clothes may start to feel uncomfortable, so choose trousers and skirts with elasticated waists. Wear loose sweaters, T-shirts or tunics on top.

Because your uterus is pressing against the bladder, you will probably feel the need to pass water urgently and frequently. Some women may need to wear an ultra-thin panty liner to catch any leaks. Your breasts will be much larger. You should be professionally fitted with a good bra in a larger back size and larger cup size.

You may be suffering from backache. This is very common during pregnancy, and is a result of your increased weight and altered posture, combined with the effect of the pregnancy hormones upon the muscles of the back. It can be a good idea to invest in a pelvic belt to give your back increased support. Practising yoga or Pilates on a regular basis can also significantly alleviate back pain, and it can often prove helpful to visit a chiropractor or osteopath.

Your heart is beating more strongly and faster than usual in order to pump an increased volume of blood around your body and into the placenta to feed the growing baby. There are more blood vessels in the vagina than before, and it will gradually become darker and softer. The nipples and surrounding areolae will be noticeably darker because of a general increase of pigmentation in your body. This increased pigmentation affects pregnant women in varying degrees, depending on their skin type and natural colouring. Women with pale skin will probably see very little change, while olive-skinned women may notice that their skin goes several shades darker everywhere, particularly around the nipples and areolae.

A dark line down the centre of the abdomen, known as the linea nigra, usually appears around the 14th week. It may be up to 1cm (½in) wide, and may stretch from the pubic hair to the navel. In some women, it reaches as far up as the breastbone. The linea nigra usually fades after delivery. If you have any birthmarks, moles or freckles, these too may darken during pregnancy.

Some women develop blotchy brown patches, called chloasma, on the face and neck. These will be intensified by the sunlight, so it is best to avoid the sun if you are affected. Chloasma usually fades after delivery, and disappears completely within around three months of the delivery of the baby.

Because of the complex hormonal changes taking place within your body, your skin may develop a healthy bloom. You can enhance this by regular walking, which will also strengthen all your muscles in preparation for labour. You may also notice how shiny and luxuriant your hair looks: this, again, happens for hormonal reasons. Once you have given birth, you will shed a lot of hair, but this is nothing to worry about.

## STRETCHMARKS

Some women develop stretchmarks on their breasts, abdomen, thighs and buttocks during pregnancy. These develop for two reasons. The extra weight and bulk you are gaining causes the collagen bundles of the skin to stretch so much that they tear. The increased levels of hormones in the blood disrupt the protein in the skin, making it thinner and more delicate than usual.

Stretchmarks show as pale wavy stripes on the skin. They tend to fade a little after the baby is delivered, but they will not disappear altogether. For this reason, it is best to do everything you can to prevent them: daily massage with vitamin E oil or essential oils, and care with your diet, may help.

Try to avoid excessive weight gain and make sure that your diet contains foods that are rich in vitamins B, C and E, as well as zinc and silica. Silica is found in wholegrains, green leafy vegetables, potatoes, nuts and seeds. A healthy diet that includes these foods will help to maintain the elasticity of your skin.

### LOOKING AFTER YOUR FEET

Your feet enlarge during pregnancy, partly because of extra fluid in the body and partly because of the extra weight you are carrying. Some women find that they go up a shoe size. The following steps will help you to care for your feet:

- Do not wear tight, rubbing footwear.
- Avoid wearing shoes with high heels while you are pregnant. A laced almost-flat shoe is the ideal choice.
- Do not wear knee-high tights (pop socks) when you are pregnant.
- Put your feet up on a footstool in the evenings. This will improve the circulation and allow any swelling to subside.
- Walk as much as and whenever you can to boost the circulation in your legs and feet.
- Avoid standing completely still, for example, when in queues. If you have to stand, keep your circulation moving by walking on the spot, and by flexing and circling your ankles.
- Have a footrest for your feet if you work for long hours at a computer or bench.

*If you work sitting down, support your legs by using a footrest; you can improvise by using a firm cushion or a pile of telephone directories.*

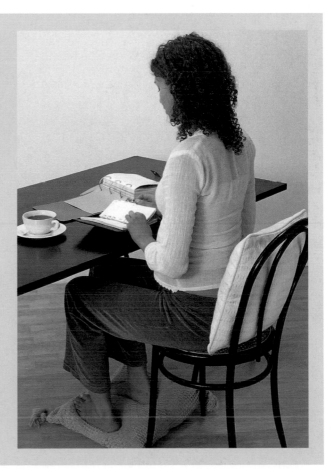

# Emotional changes

As your pregnancy progresses, you will probably experience a mixture of emotions. Pregnancy hormones are likely to make you feel more emotional and excitable than normal.

You and your partner may be growing closer together as your pregnancy advances and you become more aware of the commitment now firmly established in your lives. You are likely to be making practical plans, such as where the baby will sleep, and deciding what you need to buy and what you need to do to your home.

By now you are likely to feel more confident about your pregnancy. The chances of miscarriage are greatly reduced and the early sickness and fatigue have almost certainly eased off, leaving most women with a sense of well-being and anticipation.

However, it is very common for women to feel happy one moment, and tearful the next. Many women run the entire spectrum of emotions, from confident, optimistic and relaxed to depressed, worried, irritable and weepy. Sometimes seemingly insignificant things may set you off.

Being pregnant and anticipating your future role as a parent can bring up difficult issues from your own childhood. You may have unresolved feelings, such as sadness, anger or guilt. At the same time, you may discover insights into your parents' feelings about you.

It is important that you express your emotions and work through any unresolved issues. Talking to your partner, a close friend or relative can often be all you need. Sometimes, it may be helpful to see a counsellor or visit a complementary therapist for extra support.

## ENHANCING YOUR EMOTIONAL WELL-BEING

Most people will react positively when you tell them you are pregnant, but some may not. If someone shows a less than ecstatic response to your news, try not to let it affect you. A negative reaction is more likely to say something about that person than about your news. Some people have hidden issues about pregnancy or childbirth – for example, they may not be able to have children themselves – or they may simply not be that interested.

It can help you to deal with doubts and worries by imagining what a positive person would say if you were to ask for advice. For example, will I cope with childbirth? Well, hundreds upon thousands of women do. How will I

*Holistic therapies such as t'ai chi and yoga emphasize the importance of relaxing the body. This can help you to carry the weight of your baby more easily.*

manage without enough sleep? You will take catnaps and do less about the home than you have been used to doing. Will I be able to feed my baby? Breastfeeding does not always come naturally, but there will be people to help and advise you. At worst, the baby will not starve: you will simply bottle-feed her. There is not one problem that cannot be solved.

## TIME TO THINK

During this time, it is good to allow yourself to relax and indulge in the dreams you and your partner have for your baby. You obviously want him or her to be happy and healthy, and we all hope for a world in which our children can grow up safely.

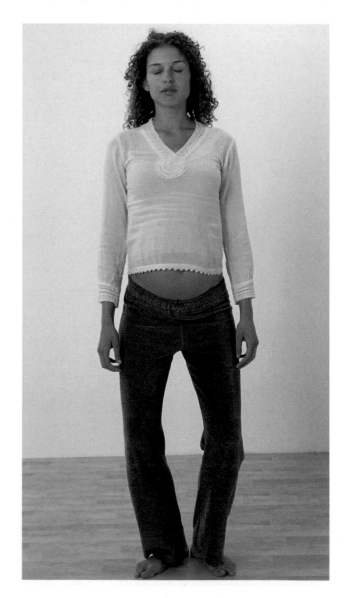

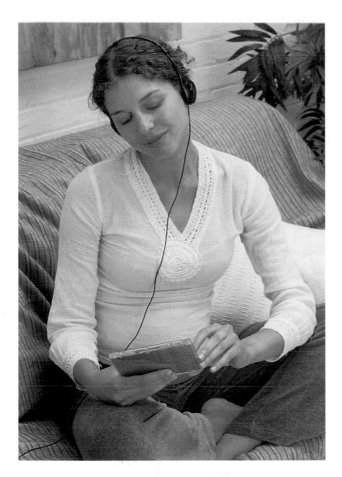

Spend time alone, just relaxing, whenever you get the chance. Enjoy listening to music, reading or simply sitting quietly and experiencing your pregnancy.

Take some time each day to allow yourself to get in touch with your feelings. Visualization can be very helpful: close your eyes and imagine the baby developing inside you. Bring to mind, too, a picture of how your own body is nurturing your growing baby.

Many parents-to-be feel that their baby is very real at this stage and begin to talk to him or her. There is good evidence to suggest that babies can learn to recognize their mother's voice before they are born. Communication need not be limited to talking. Play music, sing or stroke your belly. This can help you to form a bond long before the birth. Even if little of your communication reaches your baby, it can still have a profound effect on your emotions and enhance your psychological readiness for the most important role of your life.

## HELPING YOUR PARTNER BOND

Encourage your partner to feel your baby moving and kicking by laying his hand upon your growing abdomen. The first time that this happens can be a very exciting experience. However, it is not unusual for a father still to feel a little removed from the pregnancy at this time. Certainly all the big changes seem to be happening to

> **“** It is very common to feel happy one moment, and tearful the next. Many women run the entire spectrum of emotions during pregnancy. **”**

you rather than to him. He may even feel a little left out because of all the attention that you are attracting.

Your partner may harbour anxieties at the prospect of fatherhood, the changes it will mean for him and the changes that it will mean for your relationship. After all, you will soon be part of a family rather than a couple.

It is important that both of you have a chance to discuss your feelings, whether negative or positive. Left unspoken, they may lead to tensions in your relationship. You may be experiencing anxieties yourself about, say, the loss of freedom and your ability to accommodate both job and child. This puts you in a good position to show your partner understanding and support.

Many men do not express their feelings as freely as women. Do not worry if your partner seems to be preoccupied with readying the baby's bedroom, for example, rather than discussing his feelings with you. Be happy that actions speak louder than words.

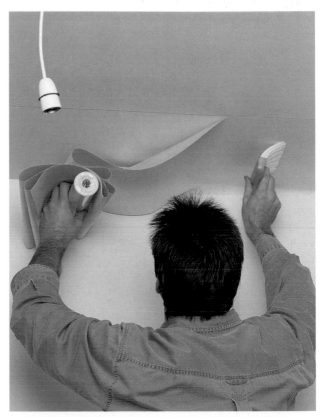

Your partner may not want to spend hours discussing the pregnancy, but may show his excitement by getting the nursery ready for your baby.

# Aromatherapy for pregnancy

It is important to take time to pamper yourself during your pregnancy. This can help you to adjust to the changes in your body, and will also enhance your emotional well-being. Aromatherapy can be an excellent feel-good therapy for the second trimester. Earlier, only a few oils are considered safe (some people think that no oils should be used), and in any case, morning sickness may make you dislike strong aromas. By 16 weeks, however, any nausea is likely to have passed and most women can use a greater range of oils.

Essential oils can be used to help alleviate a number of pregnancy-related complaints, notably stress and insomnia. They also have powerful effects on your moods. This is because scents are processed by the part of the brain that also deals with emotion and memory – making smell the most evocative of all our senses.

It is especially important that you observe basic safety precautions when using essential oils during pregnancy. Only use pure oils that you know are safe, and dilute them in a carrier oil before massaging into the skin or adding to

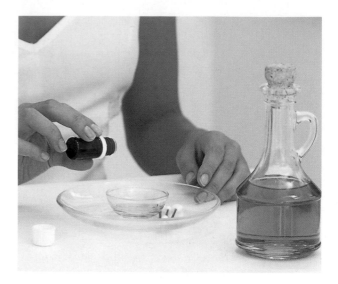

*Always dilute aromatherapy oils before you apply to the skin. Choose a good-quality carrier oil such as almond, wheatgerm or sunflower.*

the bath. Do not apply oils directly to the skin and never take them by mouth.

Many oils are not suitable for use during pregnancy; others should be used only at particular times or under the guidance of a qualified practitioner. Clary sage, for example, can be useful during labour but hazardous if used earlier. See page 149 for a list of the oils to be avoided during pregnancy. Seek professional advice if you are at all unsure about the safety of an oil.

## DILUTING AROMATHERAPY OILS

Use a low dilution of essential oils during pregnancy – no more than 1 drop per 2 teaspoons (10ml) of base oil. Use a light vegetable oil, such as sunflower or wheatgerm, as a base. If using essential oils in the bath, dilute in oil or full-fat milk, then add to a warm (not hot) bath.

Do a patch test to check for sensitivity the first time you use any oil: apply a little of the diluted mixture to your inner wrist, then wait 24 hours. If no reaction occurs, the oil is safe to use. Your skin can become more sensitive during pregnancy, so do a patch test even if you have used the oil before conceiving. Stop using any oil if you develop a reaction to it.

## USING OILS IN MASSAGE

You can use essential oils to enhance any of the massage sequences described over the following pages and elsewhere in this book. Experiment by blending different

---

### SIX GOOD OILS

Essential oils are not suitable for everyone and it is a good idea to consult a professional aromatherapist for help on choosing oils, especially if you want to treat a particular problem. The following are generally considered safe for use during pregnancy.

**ENERGIZING OILS**

- **Mandarin** Refreshing, uplifting oil made from the ripe peel of the fruit.
- **Ginger** Warming, stimulating oil that can boost the immune system. It is good used in massages or footbaths, but should not be used in the bath.
- **Petitgrain** Uplifting, sweet-smelling oil made from the leaves of the bitter orange tree (neroli is made from the flowers).

**RELAXING OILS**

- **Ylang ylang** Exotic-smelling oil that has soothing properties. It is sometimes used to help to reduce high blood pressure.
- **Neroli** Soothing oil that also lifts the spirits. It has a rejuvenating effect on the skin.
- **Lavender** Versatile oil with calming and restorative properties, which is often used to treat insomnia and stress. Can be used from 16 weeks.

---

oils together: aromatherapists use up to five but as a novice, it is probably best to use no more than two or three at a time. Relaxing blends to try after 16 weeks include neroli and lavender, or ylang ylang and sandalwood. You may like to try rosewood, a gentle, calming oil that helps to steady the emotions.

Aromatherapy massage is often recommended as a means of preventing stretchmarks, although many doctors say that massage does not make an appreciable difference. If you want to try it, use a blend of mandarin and neroli diluted in wheatgerm oil. At the very least, this will have a moisturizing effect. Adding a little avocado oil to the mixture will increase its moisturizing properties.

### OILS IN THE HOME

Use an aromatherapy oil burner to fill your home with relaxing or energizing scents. Fill the bowl with water, add a few drops of oil and heat. At night, try sandalwood, said to have aphrodisiac properties. Lavender is useful if you are having trouble sleeping (it also has antiseptic qualities). Lemon can be a good oil to burn if you are still suffering from nausea after 16 weeks.

For an aromatherapy room spray, add several drops of an essential oil to a spray gun filled with water, and spray several times around the room like an air freshener. Ylang ylang, mandarin and lavender make a refreshing blend that can help to relieve fatigue.

### IN THE BATH

Aromatherapy baths can be a great way to relax at the end of the evening: add a few drops of diluted oil to a warm bath (do not add to running water).

For a quick booster when you come home from work, try soaking your feet in an aromatic footbath for ten minutes. Two drops each of ginger and mandarin makes

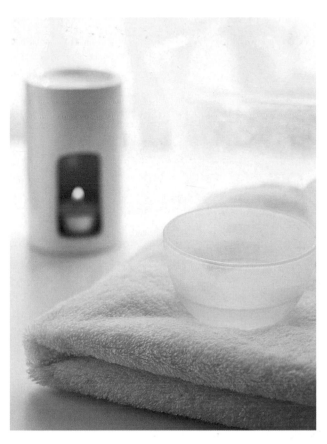

*A vaporizer offers a subtle way to experience essential oils. Try burning oils in the bedroom before you go to sleep, or in the bathroom while you enjoy a long soak.*

a warming blend, or try lavender and tea tree to soothe hot, tired feet. Add the oils, diluted in full-fat milk, to a large bowl of warm water.

To add another element to the footbath, add a large handful of marbles. As you soak your feet, roll them backwards and forwards for an easy mini-massage.

### AROMATHERAPY FIRST AID

Most of the over-the-counter remedies for colds and stuffy noses are not suitable for pregnant women, but an aromatherapy inhalation can provide effective relief. Add a couple of drops of tea tree oil to a bowl of hot water, then place a towel over your head and breathe in the aromatic steam for a few moments.

Warm aromatherapy compresses are useful for soothing general aches and pains, while a cold compress can soothe a headache or any swelling. Dilute the essential oil in full-fat milk, then add to a bowl of hot or cold water (add a few ice cubes if using cold). Drench a clean cotton cloth in the water, wring it out and then apply to the affected area.

*Try a cold lavender compress to relieve a headache, or a hot ginger compress for back pain.*

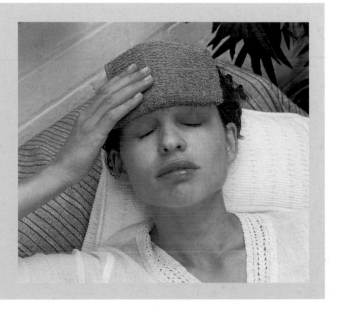

# Massage relief

We instinctively use touch to connect with each other, to nurture and to express love. This is why even the simplest form of massage can be richly comforting. Positive, gentle touch can also have a profoundly beneficial effect on our health. It is known to improve circulation, it relaxes the muscles, it helps the digestion, and it regulates the nervous system.

Massage is especially beneficial during pregnancy, provided that deep pressure is not applied to the abdomen or lower back. The number-one aim of massage is to relax mind and body, and so it can help to relieve the stresses and strains of daily living while you are pregnant. It can also help to alleviate many pregnancy-related problems, such as insomnia, circulatory disorders, high blood pressure, swollen legs and headaches.

### HAVING A PROFESSIONAL MASSAGE

A professional massage can be a real treat. Choose a qualified practitioner who is experienced in treating pregnant women (your midwife may be able to recommend someone).

Most therapists work from a consulting room, which may be in their home. Some will come to your home, particularly if you find it difficult to get around. If you are having the massage at home, make sure you heat the

> **❝ Even the simplest form of massage can be richly comforting. ❞**

room well beforehand; your body temperature will drop after you have been lying still for some time. Your masseur should bring a massage couch and towels.

Before the massage, the masseuse will check whether you have any particular aches, pains or other health problems. He or she should also ask you for a basic medical history. It is important that you tell the masseuse

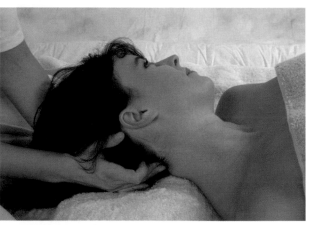

*A head massage is particularly helpful for relieving tension commonly found in the upper back, shoulders and neck areas.*

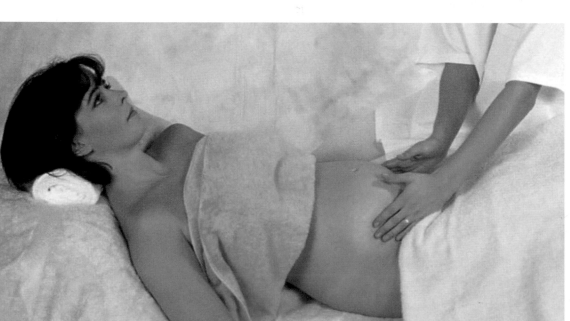

*Go to a masseuse who specializes in pregnancy and antenatal massage so that you can relax in the knowledge that you are in good hands. Enjoy.*

about your pregnancy and any health problems you have. You should tell the masseuse if you have varicose veins, since the skin over these should not be massaged.

You will be asked to undress and to lie on a massage couch, covered with a towel. You can keep your pants on if you prefer (although they may get covered in oil).

The masseuse will warm some oil in her hands and then spread it over the surface of your skin before starting the massage.

Most sessions include a full-body massage but your therapist may massage only certain areas of your body, depending on your needs. Each masseur will have a different way of combining the different massage techniques and of working around your body.

A full-body massage session usually lasts for an hour, but it may take an hour and a half if you are having a face and head massage at the same time. At the end of the session, you should be left to rest for a few minutes; close your eyes and relax. Don't plan to do anything strenuous afterwards – if possible, take the opportunity to put your feet up and relax for the rest of the day.

## SEEING AN AROMATHERAPIST

Aromatherapists work in the same way as masseurs, but they add a blend of essential oils to the massage oil. Different oils will be chosen depending on your individual needs. It is important that you like the scent of any oils used so you will be asked to smell them before they are blended together. You can also ask your aromatherapist for advice on using essential oils at home. Check that any oils used are safe in pregnancy – you should therefore see an experienced practitioner who has experience of treating pregnant women because some oils can have a harmful effect.

## MASSAGE AT HOME

You and your partner or a close friend can practise gentle massage at home. A simple massage can be a real help in soothing away general aches and in reducing tension.

Anyone can give a pleasurable massage. The key is to use slow, smooth strokes. Focus on what you are doing and ask the person you are massaging for feedback. You should not massage directly over a bone, and it is important not to apply deep pressure to the abdomen or lower back of a pregnant woman.

For a general massage, warm some oil in your hands; you want enough to give you a good slip, but not so much that your hands are dripping. Apply to the skin with plenty of smooth, stroking movements; these are very calming. Alternate between using your fingertips and whole hands. Then apply deeper pressure to release

*Ask a friend or your partner to give you a quick massage to help relieve lower back pain.*

areas of particular tension, making small circular movements with the tips of your thumbs.

It is often good to follow a back massage with a leg massage, but let your intuition guide you rather than following a set routine. Add a little more oil whenever you feel the skin starting to pull against your hands.

### Back massage

Lower back pain is probably the most common complaint of pregnancy, but a massage can do a lot to relieve the discomfort. The best way of receiving a back massage when you are pregnant is to sit astride a chair, so that you are facing its back. Lean on a cushion and drop your shoulders to help release any tension.

As well as easing your backache, a massage can also give you a comforting sense of being lovingly cared for, which is in itself beneficial. You may like to have a shoulder massage at the same time – ask the person massaging you to adapt the self-massage routine described on the following pages.

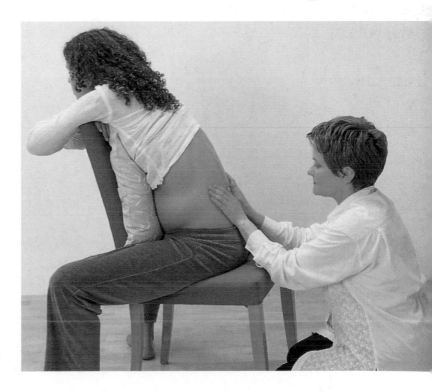

# How to massage yourself

Self-massage can be very soothing and beneficial – and you can do it whenever you like. You can use it to energize yourself before an appointment during the day or to unwind in the evening before going to bed. Massage also feels good when performed in the bath. The following routines can also be adapted for partner massage.

## Soothing tired legs

Massaging the legs is especially good if your legs ache after standing. It stimulates the circulation and soothes tiredness or swelling. Do not apply heavy pressure, and use very light movements on the inner leg.

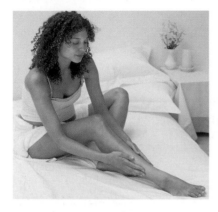

**1** Rest the foot of the leg you are working on flat, and bend the knee slightly so you can reach the lower leg. Stroke the whole leg with alternate hands, one on each side of the leg. Work up from the foot to the top of the thigh. Repeat five or six times, then work on the other leg.

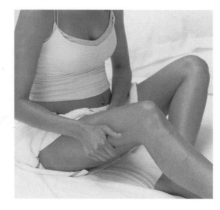

**2** Now use alternate hands to knead the thigh. Squeeze and release the flesh, working in a rhythmic fashion from just above the knee to the top of the thigh. Repeat this two or three times, and then work on the thigh of the other leg.

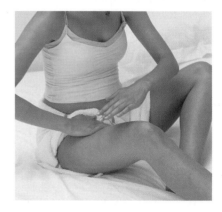

**3** Stroke the thigh, working up the thigh from the knee and using both hands, with one hand following the other. You will enjoy the smooth, flowing strokes after the more energetic kneading. Now repeat on the other leg.

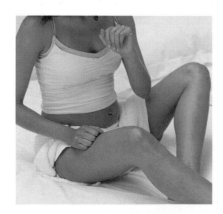

**4** Make loose fists and lightly pummel the front and outside of the thigh. This movement will help to relieve any stiffness. Pummel up the thigh a few times, and then repeat on the other thigh.

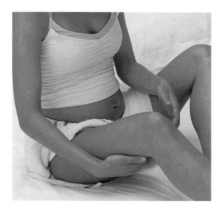

**5** Using the tips of your fingers, stroke the area around the kneecap. Hold the thigh steady with your other hand. Now stroke gently behind the knee, then continue the action up your thigh. Repeat on the other leg.

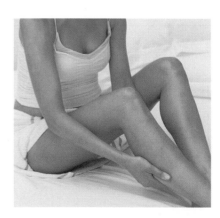

**6** Knead the calf muscle using both hands, alternately squeezing it and releasing it. Then stroke the area gently, with one hand following the other one up the back of the leg. Repeat on the other leg.

## Shoulder massage for tension-relief

Tension tends to accumulate in the shoulders, causing aching shoulders, stiff necks and headaches. This quick massage should help to relax your muscles. It is particularly beneficial if you work at a computer.

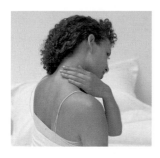 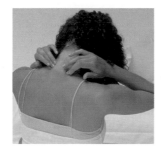 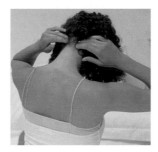 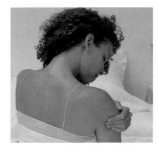

**1** Stroke the left hand down the right shoulder, working from the neck to the elbow. Do three times. Repeat on the other side.

**2** Use your fingertips to make small circles on either side of the top of the spine. Use firm but not painful pressure.

**3** Making the same circular movements, work up the neck to the base of the skull. Keep the fingers either side of the spine.

**4** Squeeze and release the flesh on your shoulder and at the top of your arm. Repeat the movements on the other shoulder.

## Feel-good facial (self-massage)

A face massage can get rid of headaches, as well as relieving fatigue and anxiety. Use a good-quality face oil to prevent any dragging of the skin. Do all the movements at least two or three times – more if you like.

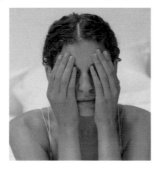 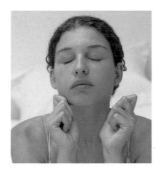 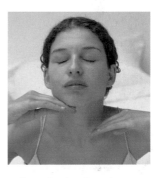

**1** Put your hands over your face, fingers on forehead. Hold for a few moments, then slowly draw them towards your ears. Do not pull the skin.

**2** Use your thumbs and the knuckles of your forefingers to inch gently along the jaw line. Begin just below the chin and work out to the ears. Pinch near the bone.

**3** Slap the backs of alternate hands under the chin. This is a good stimulating movement, and it may help to prevent a double chin.

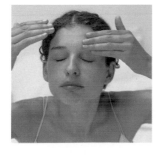 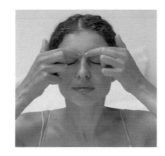 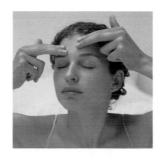 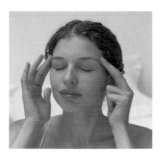

**4** Stroke your hands, one after the other, up your forehead. Work from the bridge of the nose to your hairline. Close your eyes as you do this.

**5** Place both index fingers on the bridge of your nose and stroke firmly upwards, then gently across. This may help to reduce any frown lines.

**6** Using the fingertips of your index and middle fingers, make circular movements all over the forehead. Press firmly but do not drag the skin.

**7** Using your fingertips, stroke your forehead gently, working from the centre to your temples. Finally, press them firmly against the temples.

# Treating ailments at home

Some women glow with health throughout pregnancy, but most experience minor ailments at one time or another. The majority of these health problems are not a cause for concern, but they can cause considerable discomfort. Both indigestion and constipation, for example, can be painful and irritating.

You should avoid taking medication in pregnancy if at all possible. Some natural remedies offer a safe and gentle way of relieving discomfort. They can also help to balance mood swings and strengthen the emotions.

The following remedies are generally considered safe to take during pregnancy. Even so, not every treatment will suit every pregnant woman. It is therefore a good idea to seek advice from a qualified practitioner who is experienced in treating pregnant women. You should discuss health concerns with your doctor. Always tell your doctor about any natural remedies that you are considering taking.

### HERBAL TEAS

Most herbal remedies should be taken only under the direction of a medical herbalist, but some are gentle enough to be used as self-help remedies. These include dandelion, lemon balm, meadowsweet, fennel and lime flower teas. They are available in tea-bag form from health food shops and some supermarkets, or you can make your own infusion (see box). However, do not drink herbal tea in excessive quantities – three cups a day is the usual recommended limit. Popular choices include:

- **Lemon balm or meadowsweet tea**. These can help to ease indigestion, which most pregnant women experience at some time or other. Sip a cupful after

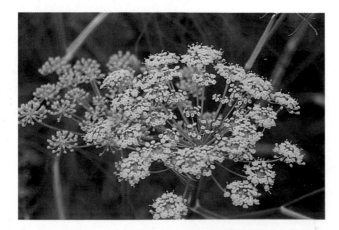

*Fennel helps with digestive problems such as constipation and also exerts a calming effect.*

each meal. Lemon balm also helps to calm the emotions, so it can be also a useful tea if you are suffering from stress or anxiety.

- **Fennel**. This is a calming herb that also works on the digestive system and acts as a mild laxative, so it can be helpful if you suffer from constipation. Infuse 5ml (1 tsp) of crushed seeds in a cup of boiling water, strain, and drink at bedtime. Drinking a cup of hot water with a slice of lemon before breakfast can also ease constipation. You should also be drinking plenty of fluid – at least eight glasses of water a day.

- **Lime (linden) flower tea**. This can help to relieve anxiety and stress, which in turn can improve your sleep. It may be helpful for stuffy noses. Chamomile is another good stress-reliever and sleep promoter.

- **Dandelion tea**. This is useful if you are feeling bloated. It works as a diuretic, so it helps to remove excess fluid from the body. It is also a good source of iron, so it can be useful if you are anaemic.

### TEAS TO AVOID

In general, do not drink one type of herbal tea repeatedly – a varied selection is key. Ask a herbalist which herbs to avoid or use in moderation during pregnancy as some encourage uterine contractions and should be avoided totally or taken only in the final stages and at the birth.

Always study the contents lists on bought teas and avoid any bought or home-made teas that contain the following: celery, cinnamon, cohosh, mugwort, nutmeg, pennyroyal and sage (sage is also to be avoided if breast-feeding). Raspberry leaf tea is a well-known uterine tonic and stimulant that helps to prepare the uterus for birth. As such, it must not be taken until the last six to eight weeks of pregnancy (one or two cups a day is a good dose) and during labour. There are many less common herbs that may be found in some teas, which is why expert advice should always be sought (see also page 148).

---

**MAKING AN INFUSION**

Place about 5ml (1 tsp) of dried herb in a cup or ceramic teapot (do not use an aluminium or tin teapot). Add a cupful of boiling water and leave to infuse for five to ten minutes. Strain, then sip slowly. To save time, make up enough for three cups and store in a vacuum flask to drink that day. Or let cool, and store in the refrigerator.

---

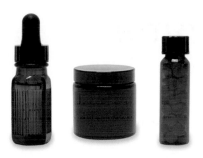

*Homeopathic remedies are usually stored in dark bottles. This helps to prevent them deteriorating.*

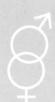
## HOMEOPATHIC REMEDIES

Natural, usually plant-based medicines, homeopathic remedies are so highly diluted that only the minutest amount of the active ingredient remains. They are generally considered very safe in pregnancy but, like any remedy, they should be used with care.

Homeopathic remedies are widely available from pharmacies and health food shops, and they are commonly used for self-help. However, it can be very difficult to choose the correct remedy for your individual circumstances without specialist knowledge. It is therefore a good idea to seek advice from a qualified, professional homeopath – who will have trained for several years – rather than trying to diagnose and prescribe for yourself. Not all women require the same remedy, even when they are suffering from what seems to be the same problem. The homeopath will also bear in mind the fact that your unborn baby is receiving treatment as well as you.

Common homeopathic remedies for pregnancy-related ailments include:

- Nux vomica, carbo veg, pulsatilla or sulphur for indigestion and heartburn.
- Aconite, belladonna, natrum mur, bryonia or sepia for headaches.
- Bryonia, natrum mur, nux vomica or sepia for constipation.
- Nux vomica, hamamelis, aesculus or sulphur for haemorrhoids.
- Calc fluor or hamamelis for varicose veins.
- Calc fluor to improve the elasticity of the skin, thus helping to prevent stretch marks.

## BACH FLOWER REMEDIES

These gentle flower- and plant-based remedies are highly diluted and are safe for use in pregnancy. They can be very helpful for dealing with difficult emotions, such as anxiety. Flower remedies are preserved in brandy, so you should take them in water. Simply add a couple of drops to a glass of water and sip throughout the day.

*Bach Flower Remedies, like homeopathic ones, are highly diluted. Just add two or three drops of your chosen remedy to a glass of water, and take sips throughout the day.*

There are 38 flower remedies to choose from. The following may be of greatest help in pregnancy:

- Olive to counteract lack of energy and fatigue.
- Walnut to help with adjusting to change.
- Red chestnut to relieve anxiety about your baby's well-being.
- Crab apple if you are feeling negative about the way that you look.
- Mimulus to help with anxiety about the birth or the effect that pregnancy is having on you.
- Rescue Remedy to use in moments of panic and general tearfulness.

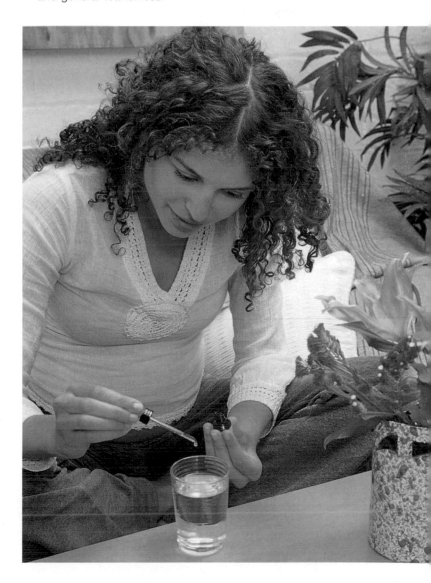

# Yoga for the second trimester

Pregnant women tend to feel more energetic and healthy in the second trimester, but the baby's increasing weight can alter your sense of balance and lead to poor posture. Yoga encourages you to stand correctly and also works to strengthen the back muscles, preventing backache. Yoga also encourages good breathing and improves the circulation, so that fresh nutritious blood reaches your baby. It is a good idea to attend specialist classes for pregnant women during the second trimester. You can also practise simple postures at home.

## Centring down

Getting your legs, rather than your lower back, to support your increasing weight and bulk is probably the most important postural adjustment that you can make during your pregnancy because it will save you from backache. Stand tall with your head erect and chin tucked in naturally. Tuck in your tail bone (coccyx). Now extend up through the spine, relaxing the tension from your upper body. At the same time, bend the knees and imagine your weight dropping downwards through the legs.

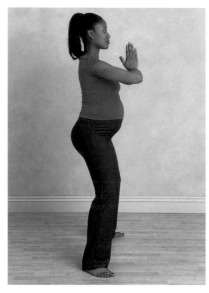

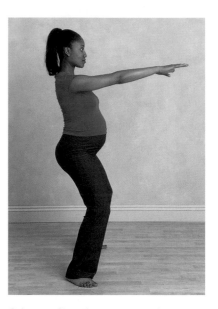

**1** Stand tall, feet apart. Bend your knees to take your weight down. Press your palms together at throat level, elbows out. Inhale, opening up your back ribs as you do so.

**2** As you breathe out, stretch your arms forwards and bend deeply in the knees. Keep your upper body erect. Hold a moment, then breathe in again. Repeat several times.

## Tiger stretch and relax

This exercise is a good way to relieve lower backache. It also helps sciatica, in which back pain extends down the leg. You will need to balance firmly on strong wrists and hands as you raise your leg parallel to the floor.

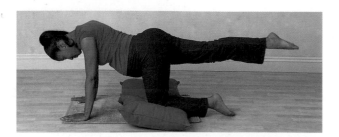

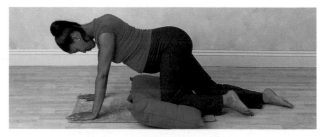

**1** Go on to all fours, with hands below your shoulders and a cushion under the knees. Extend the spine (do not dip your back). Slowly lift your right leg parallel to the floor and extend it back to release any tension. Point your toes.

**2** Let your leg sink to the floor and relax it. Maintain your balance and the strength in your spine, but drop your right hip. Shake your leg loosely from hip to toes to release pressure on the sciatic nerve. Repeat on the left.

## Swing and release

In this vigorous exercise, the palms are pressed firmly together to strengthen the arm muscles and the muscles by the upper spine. Strength in these areas makes it easier to maintain a good upright posture.

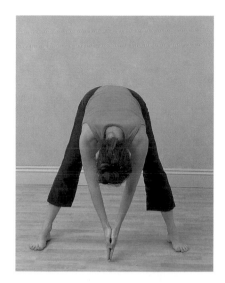 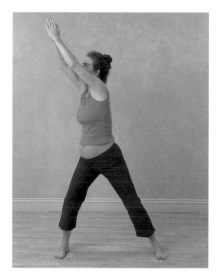 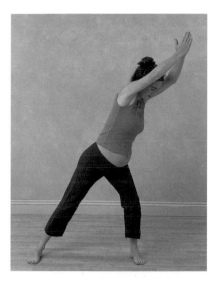

**1** Stand with your feet a comfortable width apart and your knees bent. Bring your palms together and bend forwards from the hips so that your fingertips touch the floor. Breathe out in this position.

**2** Stretch the arms forwards, pushing the palms together. Breathe in deeply, raising your head, arms and trunk up and to your right, and turning the upper body gently to your right. Hold this for a few seconds, pressing your palms together and feeling your muscles engaging along the arms and upper spine.

**3** Breathe out through the mouth, making a "HAH" sound, and drop back to the starting position with your knees bent. Keep your hands together and strong. Breathe in and out to relax in the starting position. Then breathe in again deeply to repeat the upward stretch and turn to the left. Repeat a few times.

## Modified positions for deep relaxation

It is important to relax after doing any yoga routine. As your baby grows, lying on your back will no longer be comfortable. It will also restrict circulation, so it is not a good idea, particularly from 30 weeks onwards. Instead of lying flat on your back, either bend your knees and place a cushion or blankets under your hips, lie on your side or lean forwards over a bean bag. You can even relax deeply while sitting up, as long as you are well supported and your legs are not hanging down. Take time to find a comfortable pose for you.

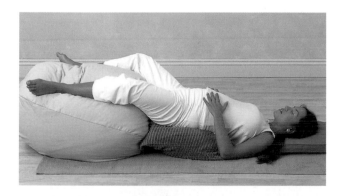

**1** Place a bean bag underneath your legs and a cushion under your hips. Your raised legs will improve the blood flow to your heart and should also reduce swelling and aching in the legs. Raising up the hips helps to take strain off the lower back.

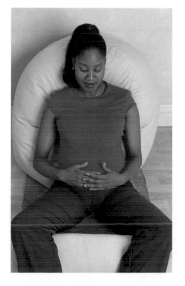

**2** Push the bean bag against a wall for extra support and recline against it so that you are as comfortable as possible. Sit with your knees bent and out to the sides and add cushions underneath to open up your hips and expand the whole pelvic area.

# Pregnancy and your sex life

The most commonly asked question about making love in pregnancy is whether or not it is safe. Experts say that it is – and there is no evidence to suggest that it might not be. A pregnancy is actually much more robust than some of us believe. Some consultants even say that it is safe to go riding – something that women are usually advised to avoid. They maintain that if the pregnancy were to be lost in this way then it was going to be lost in any case; in other words, that the pregnancy was frail. So, one need not fear causing miscarriage through the act of lovemaking.

The next big question is whether or not both you and your partner feel like making love. Some women go off sex during their pregnancy while others enjoy sex more than ever before. Similarly, some men find that their partner seems even more attractive when she is pregnant. Others are nervous of making love once their partner is visibly pregnant and prefer to wait until after the baby has arrived. However, for many couples the frequency of love-making does not change substantially whether or not the woman is pregnant.

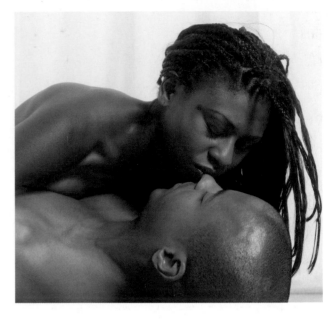

*You may find it easier to be on top when you make love with your partner, so that pressure on the abdomen is reduced and you have better control.*

If you lost interest in sex early on in your pregnancy, as many women who suffer with morning sickness do, your sex drive will probably return later on. Some women find arousal easier and orgasm more intense during pregnancy. It may be that the pregnancy hormones are responsible for this, but general feelings of well-being and happiness may also be a factor.

### GOOD POSITIONS IN PREGNANCY

Now that you are getting larger, you will probably need to experiment with different positions in which to make love. Lying on your back will probably not feel comfortable. Experiment with different positions until you find some that work well for you and your partner.

One good position to try is the spoons position, in which both partners lie on their sides. You lie with your back to your partner, who lies curled around you and facing your back. He can then enter you from behind without putting any pressure on your abdomen. You may also find it easier to use the doggy position, with you on

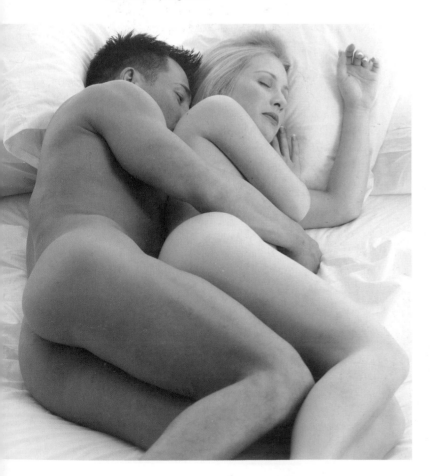

*Pregnancy can often have an impact on your sex life, but it is not necessarily a negative one. This is the time to experiment with different positions to find the most comfortable. The spoons position, where you lie with your back to your partner, is a good option.*

your hands and knees and your partner behind you. Another good position is with the woman on top, when again there is no pressure on her abdomen.

## IF YOU GO OFF SEX

If your sex drive has diminished, try to show your partner love and affection in other ways. Of course, your partner will respect your wishes but he may feel rejected or alienated all the same. Showing that you love him is all the more important at this time. Reassure him of your feelings in thoughtful ways. Give him a glorious pampering massage, cook deliciously for him, send him a card, email him during the day if he is at work.

## IF HE GOES OFF SEX

Lovemaking necessarily involves respecting one another's wishes. You may naturally find it disturbing if your partner rejects you sexually while you are pregnant, particularly if your sex life was very active beforehand. Try talking to him when he is neither tired nor busy and explain how you feel. Ask him to talk about he feels, too.

Show your partner that you cherish him in ways that are unrelated to sex. For a start, make sure that you are paying him as much attention as you are paying your pregnancy and your unborn baby. It may be that your partner has started to feel a little left out while you are, inevitably, receiving a lot of attention.

It may help if you cast your mind back to what your partner found attractive about you when you first met. Find ways to subtly recreate that picture – what did you wear? where did you go? what did you eat? You may find that focusing on your partner and his needs helps to rekindle the sexual attraction between you.

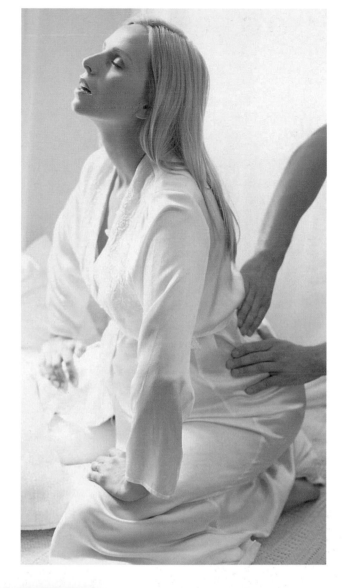

*Massage can be a wonderful way of achieving physical closeness, and relaxing together.*

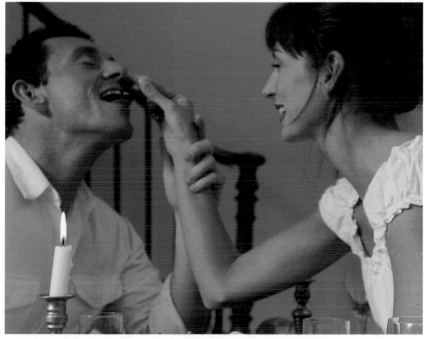

*Show your partner that you are as interested in him as ever. Make time for him and have fun together.*

# Routine antenatal care

**M**any pregnant women find that the regular monitoring and tests carried out during pregnancy cause anxiety. Sometimes the anxiety can be so great that it can outweigh the benefits of good antenatal care.

It is important to remember that antenatal care is a well-established and thoroughly researched form of preventative health, with the interests of the mother and the baby at the fore. It is now more than ten times safer to have a baby than it was 100 years ago. However, you always have the right to veto any test or procedure that you do not feel is appropriate for you.

Most women find it helpful to be fully informed and to take time to think through the significance of each test, the possible consequences and any associated risks. Make sure that you discuss any medical concerns with your family doctor or hospital consultant. You may find it useful to take notes at such consultations and discuss the matter further with your partner, a close friend or relative. If you feel unsure about any test, ask for more information and for more time in which to consider your options.

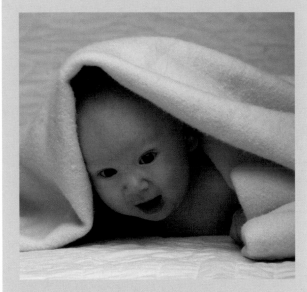

### MEDICAL TERMS
Doctors may use the following terms when talking about your baby:
- **Fetus:** 8 weeks to birth (before 8 weeks, the term is an embryo).
- **Neonate:** from birth to 4 weeks.
- **Baby:** from birth to two years.
- **Infant:** first year of life.

*The arrival of your baby may still seem a long way off, but you will soon be able to greet him or her.*

### ROUTINE MONITORING
Your weight, blood pressure, urine and blood-sugar level will be checked at antenatal appointments – changes here can give early indications of common problems.

### Weight
Your weight may be monitored throughout the pregnancy in order to judge the baby's growth, the estimated delivery date, and the amount of amniotic fluid, although very regular weight checks are now less common at many clinics as some doctors feel they are not so important. There are known disadvantages to starting a pregnancy overweight: for example, there is a stronger likelihood of pregnancy-related diabetes and high blood pressure as well as the increased risk of a difficult labour and

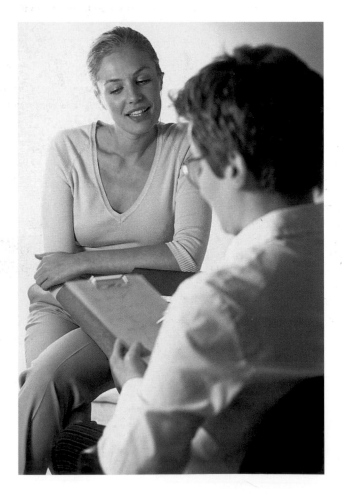

*Antenatal check-ups are a good opportunity to discuss any anxieties you may have, however small they seem.*

> **" It is now more than ten times safer to have a baby than it was 100 years ago. "**

delivering a large baby. In addition, anaesthetic complications associated with a Caesarean section are increased. These complications can sometimes occur if you gain excessive weight during your pregnancy.

### Blood pressure

Your blood pressure is checked regularly. If it is too high, it is easily brought down with medication that does not harm the developing baby. High blood pressure is a typical sign of pre-eclampsia. If left untreated, it can develop into eclampsia, which can be life-threatening to the pregnant woman and the baby. In its fully developed stage, eclampsia is characterized by high blood pressure, severe headaches and fits. The symptoms of pre-eclampsia are high blood pressure, swelling of the ankles and hands, protein in the urine and sudden weight gain.

### Urine

You will be asked to provide a urine sample at antenatal appointments. This will be checked for various substances: protein, sugar, bile, salts and blood. Urine tests are used to detect a number of conditions that could adversely affect your pregnancy, such as kidney disease, diabetes and infections in the urinary tract, such as cystitis.

For this test to be performed as efficiently as possible, you need to provide the hospital with a 'mid-stream' urine sample. To obtain this, first pass a little urine into the lavatory in the normal way, then contract your muscles to halt the flow for a couple of seconds. Resume the flow, allowing some of the urine to pass into the specimen bottle. Then remove the bottle and finish passing water.

### Blood

Your blood sugar levels are checked to see whether pregnancy diabetes has developed. Your blood may also be checked for a number of other conditions, depending upon your individual medical history.

**CHECK IT OUT**

As soon as you tell people that you are pregnant, you are likely to find yourself on the receiving end of a lot of advice, particularly from women who have already had children. It can be very helpful to talk to women who have experienced pregnancy. However, do bear in mind that antenatal procedures and our understanding of what constitutes good pregnancy care are continually changing and developing. Always check any advice with your midwife.

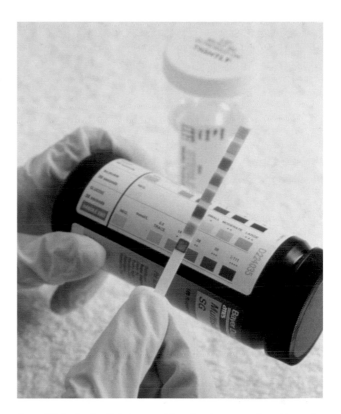

*A multiple test stick is used to check your urine at each antenatal appointment. The colour of each pad is held against a colour chart to ensure that levels of protein, blood, bilirubin, glucose, ketones and acidity are normal.*

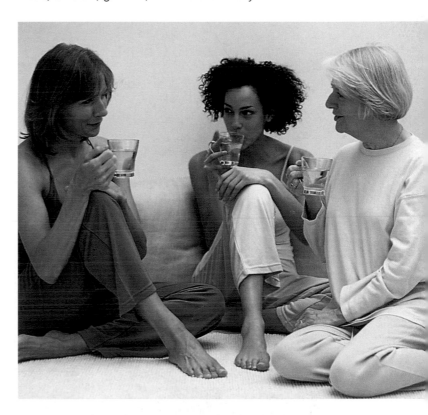

*Talking to your mother or another older woman about your pregnancy can help allay doubts and fears. However, be wary of following out-of-date advice.*

# Tests and procedures

As part of your antenatal care, you will be offered various tests to check that your baby is healthy. Some tests are standard and offered to all women; others are recommended only if the risk of a problem is higher than average. No test is compulsory: it is entirely up to you whether or not you have any procedure. However, most hospitals recommend the routine tests.

## Ultrasound

Pregnant women are usually offered their second routine ultrasound scan at around 20 weeks. This important scan is used to assess the baby's growth, to confirm the estimated date of delivery and also to check that the baby is developing in a normal way.

At the scan, the baby's head can be seen clearly in outline and its diameter can be measured on the ultrasound screen and correlated with the known average. Earlier in the pregnancy, it may be difficult to measure the head and later on, each baby will develop its own shape and size. At this point, though, most babies' heads are roughly the same size. Once the diameter of the head is measured it is plotted on a graph and equated to a known value so that an accurate estimate of the delivery date can be made.

The baby is checked in all respects including the heart, the limbs, the spine and the head, which provides the opportunity to look for any abnormalities such as spina bifida, kidney, brain and heart defects. Some defects detected at this time can be treated *in utero* (in the womb) before the baby is born. Others may require medication or surgery after the baby has been born.

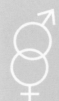

**DON'T FORGET**
The two golden rules to keep in mind when thinking about antenatal care are:
- Antenatal care is an effective and well-established form of preventative health.
- It is always your choice, for yourself and for your baby, as to which tests and procedures you do or do not have.

## Nuchal screening

This more detailed ultrasound scan is carried out between about 11 and 14 weeks, and can indicate the likelihood of a Down's baby. It is described on page 36.

## Chorionic villus sampling

This test is usually performed within the first ten or so weeks of pregnancy. It is a way of detecting the likelihood of the baby being affected by Down's. See page 36.

## Alphafetoprotein test

The substance alphafetoprotein (AFP) appears in your blood in varying levels throughout the pregnancy. Between about 15 and 18 weeks the level is fairly constant in most women (before or after this time the level is very variable). A higher than normal level at this time can indicate that the baby could be suffering from a defect of the spine, such as spina bifida, or another abnormality of brain development. A low level of AFP may be found in Down's syndrome babies.

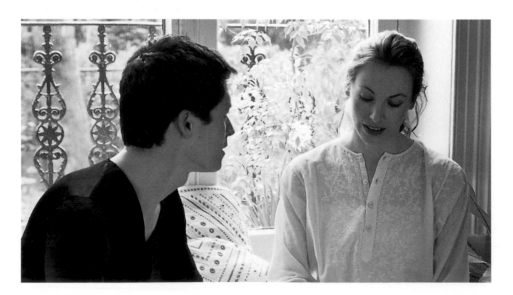

*People often have strong feelings about amniocentesis, and it is important to discuss these fully, with your partner and with the hospital consultant, before you come to a decision about the test.*

The non-invasive AFP test may be done before amniocentesis: if AFP gives a good result, you may feel that amniocentesis is unnecessary. However, AFP tests are being done less often as ultrasound can be more accurate.

### Bart's test

This test – known as the 'triple screen' in the US – involves taking a blood sample from the mother at about 16 to 18 weeks and measuring three hormones that are commonly secreted in pregnancy. The hormones are AFP, oestriol (which indicates how much oestrogen is circulating in the blood; spelled estriol in the US) and HCG (human chorionic gonadotrophin, present in high levels in pregnancy).

The Bart's test is essentially a screening test for fetal abnormality, the commonest of which is Down's. A very high result indicates the risk of a Down's child but it does not absolutely diagnose a Down's baby. The advantage with this test, like the AFP, is that it is non-invasive and you may feel it renders amniocentesis unnecessary.

### Amniocentesis

This test is usually carried out around 16 weeks. It involves a sample of fluid being drawn from the amniotic sac using a needle. Ultrasound is used to guide the needle to the correct place. The fluid is then analysed to determine the likelihood of Down's syndrome and other fetal abnormalities. The test and its implications are described in detail over the following pages.

### Fetal blood sampling (cordocentesis)

This procedure (called PUBS or Percutaneous Umbilical Blood Sampling in the US) involves taking blood from the umbilical cord and analysing the baby's blood cells. Like amniocentesis, it makes use of ultrasound to guide the needle to the correct location. Cordocentesis can be performed from the 18th week to determine the baby's condition and to identify inherited disorders such as those detected by amniocentesis.

The advantage of cordocentesis is that results are available within a week, while amniocentesis usually means a wait of up to three weeks. Cordocentesis may be used if a late ultrasound scan indicates a problem or if the alphafetoprotein test reveals a level of protein that is too low or too high. It is also useful when it is vital to know the baby's blood group before birth, as in cases of congenital forms of anaemia, or if the baby's blood needs to be tested to determine whether he or she has developed an infection – for example, of the toxoplasmosis organism.

Like amniocentesis, cordocentesis carries a small chance of causing miscarriage (it may be 1–2 per cent) – discuss this with your consultant. Rhesus-negative women will be given a protective injection of anti-D immunoglobulin after this test in case any fetal cells are disturbed, which would increase the risk of antibodies developing.

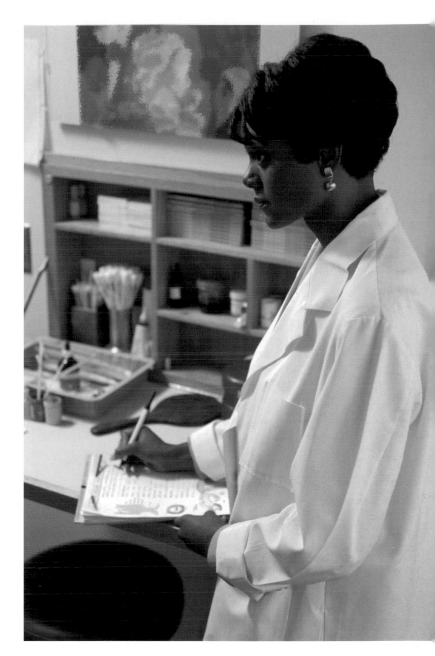

*Test samples are sent to the hospital's laboratory for analysis and interpretation. You may have to wait several weeks for some results.*

### Fetoscopy

This procedure is used only rarely and involves inserting a fibre-optic tube into the uterus through a cut in the abdomen. A microscope camera can be attached to the end of the tube so the fetus can be photographed. The fetoscope can also be used to take a sample of tissue, which enables diagnosis of several blood and skin diseases that amniocentesis cannot detect. In some centres, certain fetal conditions can be treated before delivery by means of fetoscopy. For example, babies with excess fluid of the brain can have a shunt inserted to drain the fluid. Other conditions, such as urinary tract obstruction, can be treated, too.

# Amniocentesis in perspective

Amniocentesis is an antenatal procedure that may be offered to women who have a higher than average risk of carrying a baby with an abnormality. It may be offered, for example, to women who have been in contact with the rubella virus in the first three months of their pregnancy. Amniocentesis may be offered to women in their late thirties, and will usually be offered to women over the age of forty as a matter of course.

## WHAT AMNIOCENTESIS INVOLVES

Amniocentesis is normally performed at around 16 weeks, although it can be done a little earlier and up to a few weeks later. Ultrasound is usually used to locate the amniotic sac, the placenta and the baby. It is best not to have amniocentesis without ultrasound since this increases the risk of miscarriage. In addition, the test may not be successful if insufficient liquid is obtained.

You will need to have a full bladder to have ultrasound and you will therefore be asked to drink a pint of water an hour before your appointment (and not to go to the lavatory). A local anaesthetic may be applied to your abdomen and a fine needle is then inserted through it. You may feel some discomfort at this point.

The ultrasound picture is used to locate the best pool of liquid in the amniotic sac and to make the sure that the needle does not pierce either the placenta or the baby. This is particularly important in women who are rhesus-negative as the procedure may cause the fetal and maternal blood to mix, which will sensitize the mother in future pregnancies. A protective injection of anti-D immunoglobulin is given at the time of amniocentesis to a woman who has a rhesus-negative blood group.

> " The vast majority of people are given good news after amniocentesis. "

The needle is used to draw some of the amniotic fluid. The growing baby is not harmed by the needle because it swims around in fluid and tends to move away from any object that approaches it.

After the test, it is advisable to rest for the remainder of the day in order not to irritate the uterus and to prevent leakage of fluid from the tiny hole made by the needle.

The amniotic fluid is then analysed in a number of different ways to detect fetal abnormalities. The levels of AFP hormone will also be measured. The cells will be grown (cultured) in a laboratory and their chromosomes subsequently analysed.

AFP analysis results from amniocentesis come within a couple of days but the chromosomal results of an amniocentesis normally take up to four weeks, as it takes some time to culture cells.

## IS AMNIOCENTESIS SAFE?

The main disadvantage with amniocentesis is that it carries a risk of causing miscarriage. Withdrawing the fluid can sometimes cause trauma to the uterus, which may then start contracting. Twenty years ago the risk of miscarrying a healthy baby through amniocentesis was one in 100. Improved procedures mean that it has now fallen to about one in 200.

The degree of risk depends to a certain extent on how experienced the doctor is in carrying out the technique: some doctors are more skillful than others. It also

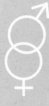

**WHO IS OFFERED AMNIOCENTESIS?**
It is up to each individual woman, in consultation with her partner, whether or not she decides to have an amniocentesis. The test will usually be offered to the following women:

- All women over the age of 37, because there is an increased risk of Down's syndrome.
- Women with a history of a child born with Down's syndrome or with certain other chromosome abnormalities.
- Women in whom a Down's blood test has shown an increased likelihood of chromosome abnormalities.

- Sometimes, women who have had a previous child affected by spina bifida or hydrocephalus. However, sophisticated ultrasound techniques may mean that an amniocentesis is not necessarily recommended in such cases.
- Women whose medical history includes having a child affected by certain sex-linked diseases, such as haemophilia.
- Certain women with a family history of rare abnormality, following genetic counselling and possibly genetic testing of several or all family members.

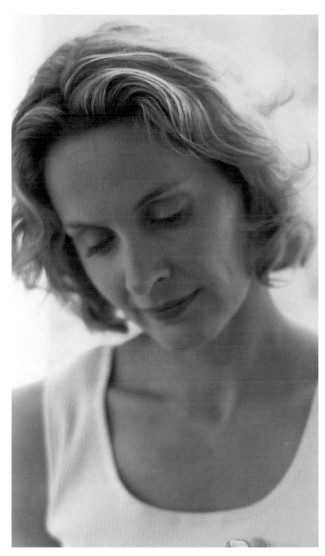

*Most hospitals will offer amniocentesis to older women, sometimes to the over-35s and usually as a matter of course to women over the age of 40.*

depends on whether or not ultrasound is used to help guide the needle. If you are considering amniocentesis, you should ask your consultant the following questions before deciding to go ahead:

- Is ultrasound going to be used?
- Who is going to carry out the test: will it be the consultant or senior registrar or another doctor?
- What is the practitioner's personal rate of miscarriage? Is it higher than the average?

When deciding whether to have the test, weigh up the risk of miscarriage against the value of the information ascertained. A 20-year-old woman has a one in 2000 chance of bearing a Down's syndrome child and a one in 200 chance of miscarriage as a direct result of amniocentesis. She is thus likely to feel that the test is not worth the risk. On the other hand, a 41-year-old woman has the same risk of miscarriage from the test, but a one in 50 risk of carrying a Down's baby. She is therefore four times as likely to have a Down's child as she is to miscarry through having amniocentesis. In this situation, many women decide that they do want to take the risk.

## THINKING AMNIOCENTESIS THROUGH

Amniocentesis is a useful test, which can offer you the peace of mind necessary to enjoy the rest of your pregnancy. It also provides valuable information for medical and nursing staff, so that they are more likely to know what, if any, abnormalities they are dealing with, and to be better prepared. The difficulties surrounding amniocentesis are:

- It could cause miscarriage and the unnecessary loss of a healthy baby.
- It could lead to a further dilemma – whether or not to terminate the pregnancy if the baby should be affected by Down's syndrome or another problem.

It is important that you and your partner share any concerns with your consultant, and ask any questions that you have before you come to a decision. Ideally, you will make a decision that all of you are happy with.

## YOUR OPTIONS

The choices you have are as follows:

- Not to have amniocentesis.
- To have amniocentesis for information, even if you are certain that you would not terminate the pregnancy if you were carrying a Down's baby.
- To have amniocentesis, having already decided that you would terminate the pregnancy in the case of a serious abnormality.
- To have amniocentesis for information, although you are uncertain as to how you would proceed in the case of an abnormality.
- To have other tests that carry a lower chance of miscarriage, in order to assess the chance of carrying a child with an abnormality. You then have the option of proceeding to amniocentesis if the risk appears to be high. Other useful tests include nuchal screening, the alphafetoprotein test and Bart's test.

## THE RESULTS

The vast majority of people are given good news after amniocentesis. The test shows that there is something wrong in about 3 per cent of cases. Nearly half of these concern Down's syndrome babies.

A termination may be recommended if the amniocentesis shows that something is severely wrong with your baby and his or her quality of life would be strongly affected. If amniocentesis identifies a less severe disability or an operable deformity, many women will continue with the pregnancy.

# When something is wrong

If tests show that something is seriously wrong with the baby you are carrying, then you will be asked if you want to end the pregnancy. Terminating a wanted pregnancy is obviously a very difficult and complex decision to make. Only you and your partner can know what is the right choice for you.

Some people feel strongly that they would not terminate a pregnancy under any circumstances. For example, people who hold profound religious or humanitarian beliefs would probably decide against termination even if there was a serious problem with the baby. Women who believe that this pregnancy is their last chance of having a child may also be reluctant to terminate the pregnancy. Some parents feel that they are able and willing to care for a disabled child, whatever the extent of his or her problems.

Many couples would, however, consider termination the most feasible option if a test such as amniocentesis or chorionic villus sampling (CVS) showed that the baby was not developing normally. There are many reasons why a pregnancy may be terminated. These are just some of the common ones:

- The parents may know that they could not cope with a disabled child.
- The parents may believe it to be wrong to bring a child into the world if she or he would develop an incurable, untreatable disease.
- The mother's physical and mental well-being may be at risk. If the child is so severely handicapped that he or she will inevitably die later in the uterus or shortly after birth, the mother, and the father, may be saved some suffering by opting for a termination.
- The likely effect on the parents and other children in the family may seem too great. A severely handicapped child can exert a profound influence upon its family. He or she will need full-time care and this may strain the emotional, physical and financial resources of the family to a great degree.
- The child may suffer needlessly and die either in childhood or in early adulthood.

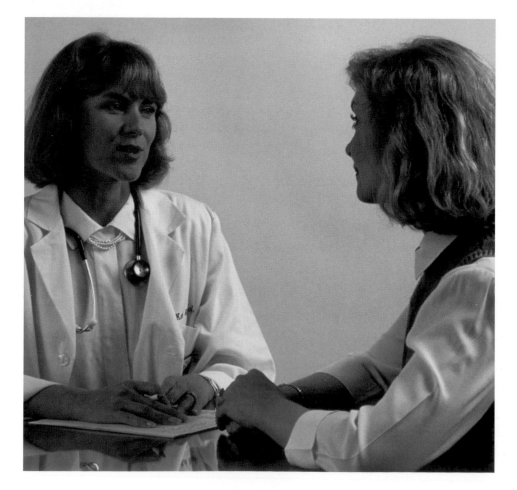

*Everyone involved in maternity care knows that choosing to have a termination is the most distressing decision a woman can make. You will be given all the support that you need.*

You may want to talk to your family doctor, the hospital consultant or your midwife more than once if you are contemplating a termination. Healthcare staff will understand only too well that you need to gather as much information as possible, and that you need to take time to make your decision. Rest assured that nobody will try to persuade you to have a termination if you really do not wish to do so.

## TERMINATING A PREGNANCY

The procedure for terminating a pregnancy varies depending on whether it is performed before the end of the 13th week or after it. If you are considering having a termination after an amniocentesis, you will need to have a late termination.

### Early termination

A termination performed at 13 weeks or earlier is a simple and quick operation, with minimal risks to the woman's physical health. It may be done following a test carried out early in the pregnancy, such as CVS.

Early terminations are carried out under general anaesthetic. The woman's cervix is dilated (expanded) so that the fetus can be removed by suction. You will usually be able to go home on the same day as the operation, but you will be advised to rest for 24 hours.

### Late termination

A late termination is available to those women who wish to end a pregnancy after amniocentesis or other tests. At this stage of pregnancy, it is not possible to dilate the woman's cervix to the required degree without risking permanent damage to it. Because of this, many doctors prefer to use the technique in which the natural process of birth is imitated.

The woman is given synthetic prostaglandin in the form of a vaginal gel or pessary, or in the form of an infusion directly into her uterus, at regular intervals. This process is known as prostaglandin induction, and causes the woman to go through what is, in effect, a mini-labour. Her uterus starts contracting to expel the fetus, and in response to this, the cervix dilates. If the pregnancy is being terminated after 20 weeks, then an irritant substance may be injected directly into the amniotic sac around the fetus.

It may be some hours before the fetus is expelled, just as it is during labour and birth. The fetus is usually born dead. The woman then normally undergoes a procedure called dilatation and curettage (D and C) in which all the contents of the uterus are removed. This is done to ensure that no part of the placenta or anything else relating to the pregnancy remains.

You will probably have to stay in hospital overnight, and should rest at home over the days that follow.

## THE RISKS

There are certain risks attached to terminating a pregnancy, and these risks are higher the later the abortion. Your doctor will explain these to you in detail, but they include:

- Infection in about 3 in 100 women.
- Prolonged bleeding in 4 in 100 women.
- Abnormal blood clotting in one in 200 women.
- Operative trauma, such as tissue damage or perforation of the uterus. This occurs in less than one in 100 women.
- Feelings of regret for what might have been. Most women will need time to come to terms with the end of a wanted pregnancy.

## FEELINGS OF REGRET

In cases where the developing baby has, or is likely to have, severe abnormalities, having a termination may be the best choice for everyone. However, this does not mean that you will not mourn your baby. Ultimately, this may prove to be an event in your life that is never completely forgotten, never completely accepted.

It is extremely important that, immediately after the event, you give yourself whatever time you need to grieve and to fully explore and express your emotions. Talk to your partner about how you feel, and also encourage him to share his feelings.

You may wish to carry out some kind of closing ceremony or ritual to help you say goodbye. How you choose to do this is a personal matter, but you could visit a local church or religious centre of some kind, or simply go somewhere beautiful and say goodbye in your own way. Making a donation to a children's charity or perhaps planting a tree that will live for many years may feel like a positive and helpful thing to do.

## FINDING SUPPORT

You and your partner may well need support from other people – don't feel that you have to sort out your feelings between just the two of you. Friends and relatives can be a great source of comfort, although they may be too close to the two of you and to the situation. If you prefer to see a counsellor, your family doctor will be able to refer you. There are centres you can contact direct that offer specialist post-termination counselling and also confidential helplines. Remember that such counsellors are happy to discuss your feelings about a termination even if it is years after the event.

A complementary therapist may also be able to offer support. Acupuncture and zero balancing – a therapy in which gentle touch is used to release difficult emotions – may go some way towards helping you to deal with what has happened to you. Reiki is another gentle and non-intrusive method of healing that might prove helpful.

# Checklist of common problems

By the second trimester, women usually feel healthier and more confident about their pregnancies. You are likely to have more energy, and morning sickness has usually passed. However, you may still be affected by ailments such as constipation and indigestion.

The following solutions should help to relieve any discomfort, but also check the relevant safety advice in Chapter Six.

Some treatments may work better for you than others and you may need to experiment to find one that suits you. If any complaint persists, or if it troubles you, or you are not sure what it is, you should consult your family doctor. In any case, tell your midwife about the problem at your next antenatal check.

**Back pain** Many women suffer from back pain during pregnancy (and almost everyone is affected in the last months). However, there is a lot you can do to minimize the pain. First of all, make sure that you have a good, supportive mattress; if you do not, consider buying a new one. Be aware of your posture: check how you are holding yourself at regular intervals, and change your position if you are sitting awkwardly. Try yoga or Pilates, which can help to strengthen the muscles in your back and improve your posture.

For persistent back pain, see an osteopath, Alexander technique teacher or chiropractor. Flotation therapy, which allows you to relax in a supported position, can be a pleasing way to relieve back pain. Reiki, massage and acupuncture can also be good therapies to try.

**Varicose veins** Eat a healthy diet, that includes plenty of foods that are rich in vitamin E, such as wheatgerm, wholegrains, sunflower seeds and cold-pressed vegetable oils. Avoid standing still for long periods: walk on the spot or flex and rotate your ankles. Walk daily to help the circulation, and rest with your feet up twice a day, for 20 minutes a time. Brushing the skin daily with a soft-bristled brush can help – use long, upward strokes.

For temporary relief, apply commercially prepared witch hazel or aloe vera compresses to the affected area. Ask your doctor about wearing support stockings. Homeopathy, acupuncture and aromatherapy can be helpful. You may also draw comfort from the fact that varicose veins often subside after the birth.

**Stretchmarks** Eating a healthy, balanced diet that is rich in vitamin E, silica and other nutrients can help to

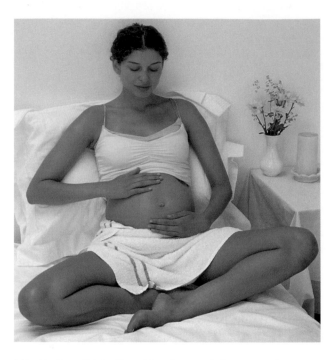

*Massaging oil into the skin of your abdomen, using a circular clockwise motion, may help to prevent the formation of stretchmarks.*

prevent stretchmarks (see also page 51). Massage the skin gently with a good-quality oil enriched with vitamin E to help maintain suppleness. Add a few drops of an essential oil such as neroli or mandarin to your massage oil. Marigold or lavender flowers can also be used. Soak the flowers in wheatgerm oil for two weeks, then strain. Apply the oil daily, rubbing it gently into the skin in a circular motion. A homeopath may prescribe calc fluor as a preventative measure.

**Constipation** Start the day with a glass of hot water with a little fresh lemon juice. Include plenty of wholegrains, fruit and vegetables in your diet, and drink lots of water. Avoid bananas and hard-boiled eggs, and do not eat late at night. Take more exercise, particularly walking, and try yoga – some yoga postures specifically work on the digestion.

For temporary relief, try massaging the abdomen with essential oil of ginger diluted in wheatgerm oil (see pages 54–7): use a smooth circular movement, starting on the lower left-hand side and working clockwise (apply light pressure only). Herbal medicine, homeopathy, acupuncture, chiropractic and osteopathy can all be helpful.

**Haemorrhoids** Piles are often caused by constipation, so follow the steps given. Try resting on your left side regularly; this can relieve pressure on the pelvic veins. Keep the area clean, washing with unperfumed soap after emptying your bowels. Cold, witch hazel compresses can help relieve itching. However, be sure to tell your doctor or midwife about the problem.

**Headaches and migraines** Eat regularly and make sure that you are drinking enough water – low blood sugar and dehydration can lead to headaches. Try to identify any migraine triggers, such as cheese, chocolate, citrus fruits and caffeine, and avoid them. Watch your posture: relax your shoulders regularly since tension here can cause headaches. A shoulder massage can provide temporary relief, as can applying a lavender-oil compress to your temples. Consider seeing an Alexander technique teacher, chiropractor, osteopath or cranial osteopath. Reiki, reflexology and acupuncture can also help.

**Cystitis** Urinary infections require immediate treatment: see your doctor if you have an increased need to pass urine, and burning or pain when you do so. Drinking plenty of water and two glasses of cranberry juice a day will help prevent and ease cystitis. Tea tree and lavender oils have a healing effect: dilute two drops of each in a base oil or full-fat milk and add to a warm bath. Do not use lavender if you are less than 16 weeks pregnant.

A homeopath may recommend remedies such as cantharis or apis mel, which can be taken alongside antibiotics. Reflexology and herbal medicine can also be useful as an adjunct to medical treatment.

**Thrush** See your doctor to check the diagnosis, even if you have had thrush before (other vaginal infections may also cause itching, redness and discharge). Many women

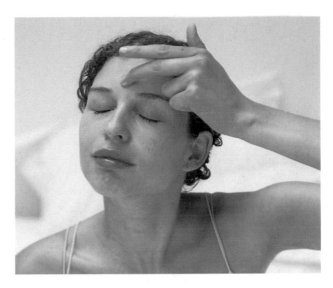

*You may be able to relieve a headache by massaging the acupuncture points just above the bridge of the nose and at the external tip of each eyebrow.*

find that it helps to avoid sugar and yeast, and to eat plenty of vegetables. You should make sure that you use unscented soap and bath products.

Live yogurt is a soothing natural remedy: apply to the affected area every two hours. Tea tree and lavender essential oils may help: try diluting two drops of each in a base oil or full-fat milk, and add to a warm bath. If you are less than 16 weeks pregnant, use tea tree oil only.

**Indigestion** Eat little and often rather than having two large meals a day. Limit fluid intake at mealtimes, and eat slowly. Do not bend or lie down afterwards, and make sure that you eat your evening meal at least two hours before bedtime. If indigestion persists at night, use more pillows to keep your upper body elevated. Try drinking lemon balm tea after meals, and ask your doctor about taking calcium-based indigestion tablets. Homeopathy, acupuncture, osteopathy, Alexander technique and chiropractic can all be beneficial.

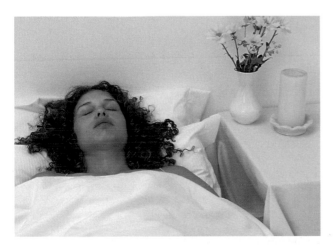

*If you suffer from heartburn at night, do not sleep on your back; sleep on your side propped up with pillows. Do not eat less than two hours before bedtime.*

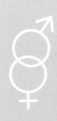

**WHEN TO CALL A DOCTOR**
Seek emergency assistance if you have:
- Vaginal bleeding other than spotting.
- Severe abdominal pain or vomiting.
- Sudden swelling of hands and ankles or blurred vision with severe headache.
- From week 22, no fetal movements for more than 12 hours.
- Breaking of the waters.

See your doctor if you have:
- A high temperature (101°F/38.5°C +).
- Swollen hands or ankles.
- Pain on urination.

# Common Qs and As

**Q**: I am getting irritated by all the advice that I am receiving from anyone and everyone, and by all the tests that one is given during antenatal care. Is all this fuss necessary?

**A**: It is important to distinguish between well-meant advice from friends and family, and that from your doctor and midwife. Remember that friends and family may not be up to date – some of what you are told may not be correct. Antenatal care, however, is valuable. Today, it is the expectation of most women in the West that they will have a safe and successful pregnancy leading to the delivery of a healthy baby. This is in stark contrast to our grandmothers and great-grandmothers. Before 1935, one in every 200–250 pregnancies resulted in the death of the mother, most commonly from infection. These days you almost never hear of women dying in childbirth – thanks largely to regular antenatal monitoring and improved delivery procedures.

**Q**: My sister has been trying for a baby for three years. Now that I am pregnant she is avoiding me. What can I do?

**A**: This is a very difficult situation, particularly for your sister. It may help to be open about what is happening; perhaps you could tell her that you fully realize how painful it is for her to be around you while you are pregnant and that you understand how she is behaving. You could also reassure her that many couples do conceive after several years of trying, and encourage her to see her doctor for investigations if she has not already done so.

You may want and need your sister's support at this eventful time in your life, but it is probably best to let her decide how much she wants to be involved with your pregnancy. If she does remain distant, you may find that the situation changes when the baby is born, and your sister can enjoy her niece or nephew.

**Q**: How would I know if there was anything wrong with my baby?

**A**: The chief way of checking that everything is progressing well is through your regular antenatal checks: this is why it is so important that you attend them. If anything should be amiss, it can be quickly identified and treated.

If there were anything seriously wrong, your body would soon tell you. Be alert to the chief danger signs and symptoms, which are listed on page 75. Be aware, too, of your baby's movements. Should these stop for a period of 24 hours or more, you should consult a doctor without delay.

**Q**: I am five months pregnant and have only a very small bump. Is something wrong?

**A**: Women do vary in the size of their bump, and if you are of a slight build you are more likely to give birth to a baby who also has a slighter build. However, if you are worried, the best thing for you to do is to talk about your concerns with your antenatal team. They should be able to reassure you that everything is fine.

One of the great advantages of antenatal care and all the research that has gone before is that the hospital consultants will almost certainly know if anything is wrong. They will be able to tell if you are carrying what is known as a 'small for dates' baby. They will also know from blood and urine tests, as well as from the scans, if the pregnancy is not progressing as it should do.

Q: I feel uncomfortable about the whole idea of making love now that I am well into the pregnancy, and worry that some damage may be done. Am I being ridiculous? Exactly how safe is it?

A: There are certain circumstances under which sex must be avoided – in certain high-risk pregnancies or in the last trimester when expecting more than one baby, for example. Your doctor will advise and warn about this. However, in the majority of cases, experts feel that there is no danger at all in making love at any stage of the pregnancy, as long as you are not overly athletic.

You will find that you need to explore different positions as your size increases, in order to be as comfortable as possible. Also, be prepared for some loss of libido at certain stages due to hormonal changes or fatigue. Take time to explore non-penetrative options and always keep loving lines of communication open with your partner.

Q: I cannot decide whether or not to have an amniocentesis. I would be devastated if I lost the baby through having the test.

A: This is without doubt an extraordinarily difficult decision to make. You should discuss with your hospital consultant the risks of your particular case, bearing in mind your medical history and your age. Then give yourself and your partner time to consider how much you are personally at risk of carrying a baby with a serious problem such as Down's syndrome. If the risk is slight, you may be well advised not to have amniocentesis. If the risk is thought to be high or very high, you may prefer to have the test. However, if you knew that you would be devastated at the loss of any baby, whether or not he or she was impaired with a condition such as Down's, clearly it would be better if you did not have the test.

Q: If I had to terminate a pregnancy, how long would I have to wait before we started trying for another baby?

A: Medical opinion remains divided on this issue. The minimum wait is naturally until your periods return to normal or at least return to what was normal for you. After that, the general consensus is that you should wait for three or four months before attempting to conceive again. If you wait a little longer than that, both you and your partner will have that little extra time in which to recover both physically and emotionally after the termination. Some consultants advise six months but this is not strictly necessary.

Q: My doctor says that I need a course of antibiotics to clear up a severe attack of sinusitis. I am worried about taking medication when I am pregnant. Do you think that it is okay to take them?

A: You should obviously avoid taking any unnecessary medication during pregnancy. However, if the infection is severe, clearly it needs to be treated before it starts to affect your general health and energy levels. Any medication prescribed during your pregnancy will be given in the knowledge that you are pregnant and will be chosen accordingly. Always remind any prescribing doctor that you are pregnant, just in case he or she fails to refer to your notes and especially if you are not yet big enough for it to be obvious.

# CHAPTER THREE
# The third trimester

" It is important for you to make rest and relaxation a priority. "

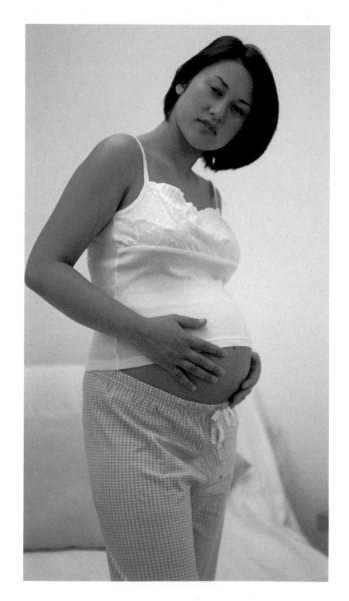

You are now embarking on the last trimester of your pregnancy, week 27 onwards. This is a tumultuous, exciting time for you and your partner. Now that your baby is fully formed, you may more easily be able to imagine him or her as a little person.

The normal length of time for a pregnancy is 40 weeks, but yours may last just 38 – less if the baby is premature – or it may run to 42. Once a pregnancy goes beyond 42 weeks, medical intervention may be recommended. If you are pregnant with twins (or more), you will almost certainly deliver early, usually at about 37 weeks.

During these last weeks, you may feel that you have been pregnant forever. You may feel slightly breathless when bending down. Your sleep may be interrupted when you turn over, by frequent trips to the lavatory, and by kicks from your baby.

It is important for you to make rest and relaxation a priority. Take a rest every day, and perhaps chat to

*You may feel a greater bond with your baby in these last weeks. Now you can start looking forward to getting to know him or her in person.*

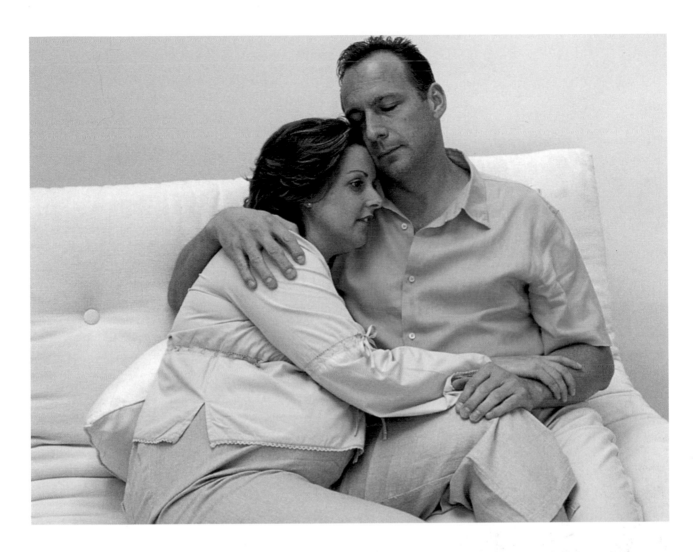

your baby or play music as you do so. Complementary therapies can be particularly beneficial during the last three months. Good ones to try include reiki, yoga, massage, aromatherapy and Alexander technique. These will encourage you to relax, improve your posture and help relieve any backache that you may be experiencing.

Do not attempt to do any more than you feel comfortable with, but remember the value of exercise. A short walk each day will improve muscular fitness and at the same time boost your energy and prepare you for labour and the birth.

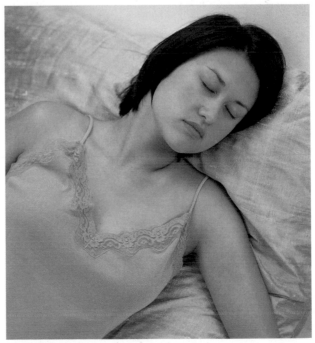

*Top: You may feel increasingly disinclined to go out as your pregnancy progresses. Spending quiet evenings at home with your partner can seem far more appealing.*

*Sleep may become more fitful in later months. Get as much relaxation as you can, and take an afternoon nap to compensate if possible.*

# How your baby is developing

uring these last months of your pregnancy, the baby will continue to mature, and he or she will also become much fatter.

### Weeks 26–27

The eyelids open briefly for the first time at the end of the second trimester; they start to remain open from week 27. The iris of the eye is blue at this stage, and will remain so until a few months after delivery. The baby looks quite lean, and at 26 weeks weighs about 500g (1lb 2oz). Over the next few weeks, his or her body weight will more than double as more muscle and fat develops.

### Weeks 28–31

At 28 weeks the baby measures 36cm (14in), and weighs about 900g (2lb). You will feel a good deal of kicking and fluttering at this stage. Your baby's breathing movements will have become rhythmic by week 30, but he or she may experience hiccups – which you will feel as small jerks – when amniotic fluid goes down the wrong passage.

If your baby were to be born at this point, there is a fair chance that he or she would survive. However, the lack of body fat means that the baby would have difficulty in regulating his or her body temperature. He or she would also experience breathing difficulties and would need to be placed in an incubator with a ventilator attached. The baby's immune system and liver functioning would still be weak, rendering him or her particularly susceptible to infection. Specialist care would be needed for several more weeks while the baby continued his or her development outside the uterus.

### Week 32

Your baby is perfectly formed, with fully developed lungs. It has been shown experimentally that the baby can now focus on external stimuli – a needle, for example. From now until week 34, your baby is likely to turn so that he or she is head down, in preparation for the birth. Before this time most babies are in the breech position, with the head facing up. The baby weighs about 1.8kg (4lb).

## THE FINAL STAGES

You will become much larger in the last trimester as your baby is growing rapidly. Your expanding uterus will press against your intestines and stomach, impeding your digestion, and on the lungs, causing slight breathlessness. The baby is fully formed at 36 weeks but needs to put on weight before birth.

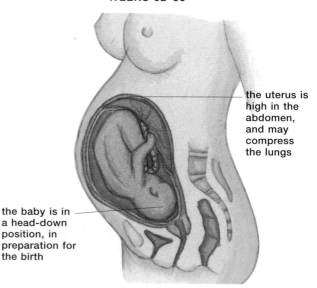

**WEEKS 27–31**

the uterus expands upwards as well as outwards

the baby has room to manoeuvre from side to side

*By about week 27, your expanding uterus is halfway between your navel and ribs.*

**WEEKS 32–36**

the uterus is high in the abdomen, and may compress the lungs

the baby is in a head-down position, in preparation for the birth

*Between weeks 32 and 36, the uterus has expanded to fill the abdomen, extending almost up to the ribs.*

## Weeks 33–36

The baby is becoming plumper and gaining about 14g (½oz) of fat each day. Fat ensures that a baby can regulate heat and cold once they leave the controlled environment of the uterus. The fingers and toes have soft nails, which reach right to the ends. The hair on the baby's head may be as long as 2.5cm (1in) long and is very slippery to aid the baby's passage during birth. By week 36, the baby's skull is firm but not hard, because it will need to compress as the baby squeezes down the birth canal.

The baby is about 46cm (18in) long and weighs about 2.75kg (6lb). If this is your first baby, the head will soon engage – drop downwards into the upper pelvis – in preparation for the birth. If you have given birth before, the baby may not engage for several more weeks, and sometimes not until just before the labour.

## Weeks 37–39

Your baby's nervous system is maturing, ready for birth. The layer of fat under the skin is now ready to regulate body temperature when the baby is born. The lungs are lined with surfactant, which resembles bubbles of foam. This keeps the lungs partially inflated each time the baby breathes out after she is born; without surfactant the lungs would collapse. The baby's heartbeat is about twice as fast as yours, about 110–150 beats per minute.

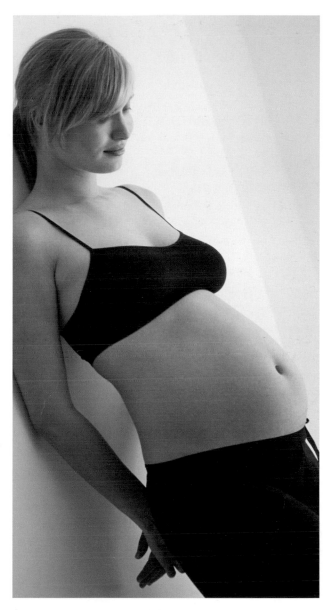

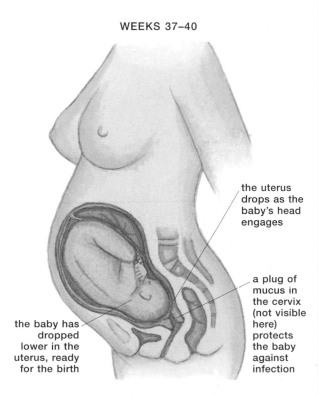

WEEKS 37–40

the uterus drops as the baby's head engages

a plug of mucus in the cervix (not visible here) protects the baby against infection

the baby has dropped lower in the uterus, ready for the birth

*Some time from week 36 onwards, the head engages. The uterus drops lower, easing pressure on the lungs.*

*During these final weeks, you will feel a variety of movements as your baby turns over, moves his or her hands and feet, and even hiccups. These movements are often felt more when you are resting.*

Other people may now be able to hear the baby's heartbeat simply by putting their ear to your abdomen. The baby will weigh about 3.1kg (almost 7lb).

## Week 40

The baby's movements decrease from now on, because there is less space in the uterus for him or her to move around. You may miss these movements, although you may still feel strong kicks from the baby's hands and feet. When the baby is awake, his or her eyes are open a good deal of the time. In a boy, the testicles will almost certainly have descended. The baby may now measure about 51cm (20in) in length and he or she weighs about 3.5kg (7lb 8oz).

# How your body is changing

You will experience both physical and emotional changes in the last three months. The often powerful emotions are nature's way of preparing you for all the changes and challenges ahead. Heightened sensitivity and the ease with which tears often flow are all signs that you are in an emotional state that will make you peculiarly responsive to your newborn baby. In this way nature ensures that you look after your baby, that you respond to cries, that you feed him or her, and that you keep the baby with you and protect him or her from others.

You and your partner may watch, curiously, as your body steadily changes in shape and size. During the third trimester, the changes become much more pronounced.

There are five principal signs that help to indicate that your baby is well and progressing normally towards delivery. These signs are:

### The baby's kicks

You will feel a lot of kicking. Many babies are lively at certain times of day, suggesting that they develop a regular pattern of sleep and activity. Babies are often most active when the mother is resting.

### Breathlessness

It is common to be out of breath in pregnancy, particularly in the last few weeks. You may feel quite short of breath

*Towards the end of your pregnancy, Braxton Hicks contractions can cause discomfort, but they do not last long. Unlike labour contractions, they are irregular and do not increase in intensity. Putting your hands on your belly and breathing deeply may help to relieve them, and they usually stop if you have a bath or lie down.*

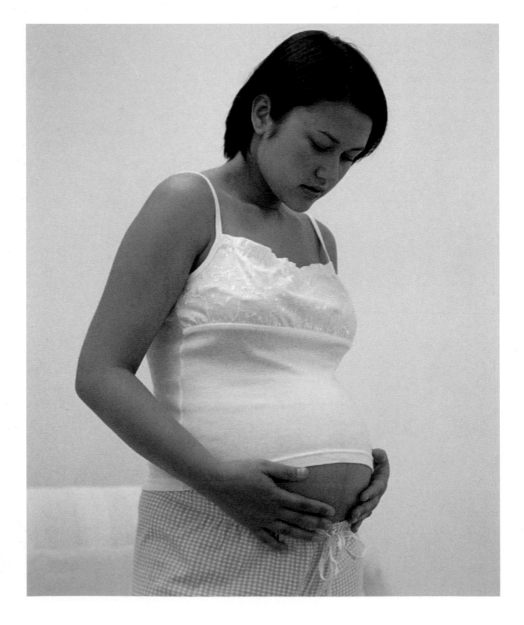

during even relatively minor exertion. This happens for two reasons. Your lungs are working twice as hard as usual in order to supply both you and the baby with oxygen, and the work of the lungs has been made harder because the baby is now so large that he or she is pressing up against your lungs. Rest assured that the baby will receive enough oxygen, even though you may sometimes find yourself panting with the effort.

### Increased urine frequency

You will probably want to pass water often, and you may be caught short now and again. This happens partly because the baby is pressing upon all your internal organs, including your bladder, and partly because your muscles have become smoother and softer, in preparation for the birth, when they will be required to stretch to the limit. When you urinate normally, you relax your muscles. When you are pregnant, these muscles tend to relax of their own accord whether you want them to or not. That's what causes the feeling that you need to pass water, and what can cause slight incontinence, too.

### Small and irregular contractions

'False labour' contractions can start from week 23, or even earlier, although some women do not experience them at all. They feel like a tightening in the abdominal area. Towards the end of pregnancy, these contractions are known as Braxton Hicks contractions and they become more pronounced, although they are still nothing like the contractions for labour. These 'false labour' contractions last for no more than 20 seconds or so.

When you go into labour, contractions will be more powerful and last for 40 seconds or more. Some specialists maintain that contractions occur throughout pregnancy in order to encourage the blood flow in the placenta, which brings oxygen to the baby.

### Engagement

The baby's head becomes engaged in the upper part of the pelvis, usually after the 36th week. All through pregnancy, your uterus expands upwards in your body in order to accommodate the baby's increasing size. The baby is quite low down in your body during the first trimester; after this, he or she rises steadily upwards until week 36. Then, the lower part of the uterus expands, in preparation for the baby's birth, and the baby moves downwards a little.

The baby's head engages in the upper part of the pelvis ready for delivery just a few weeks later. You will experience this as pressure against the cervix (the neck of the uterus). Women who have had babies before may find that their baby's head does not engage so soon, not until the final week of the pregnancy or even as late as the start of labour.

Your increasing size and the frequent activity of the baby mean that you may need extra support to keep you feeling well. Natural therapies can be really helpful in relieving any sleeplessness, stress, tension, fatigue and anxiety that you might be experiencing. They can also help you to feel good about yourself, encouraging you to revel in your swelling size – after all, this is a sure sign that your baby is progressing well.

### SUPPORTIVE NATURAL THERAPIES

A weekly session with an experienced therapist may help you cope better with the ups and downs that are often part of pregnancy. Acupuncture, aromatherapy massage and reflexology can all help you to maintain a sense of balance and well-being.

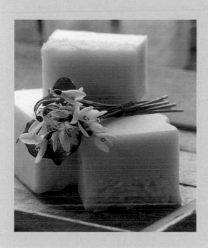

*Small feel-good treats – such as soaps scented with essential oils, or gentle herbal home treatments – can lift your mood and relieve tension in the last weeks.*

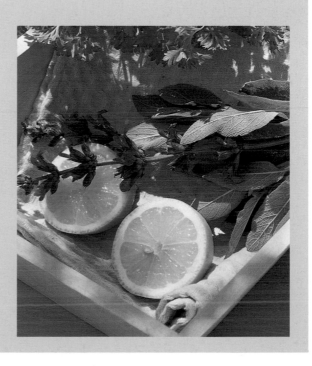

# Emotional changes

The last few months of pregnancy are a time of great anticipation and preparation. Both emotionally and mentally, you are readying yourself to become a parent. Physically, your body is gearing up for the birth as well as meeting the needs of your rapidly growing baby. On a practical level, you are likely to feel a strong urge to create a welcoming home for your child.

Not surprisingly, many women find that they become more inward-looking during the third trimester. You may feel absent-minded or forgetful, or rather detached from the world. Work, family and socializing may become less important to you as your focus turns towards the birth.

However keen you are to have your baby, you may experience a real sense of boredom about the pregnancy, particularly in the last weeks. It may feel as though you have been pregnant forever. Now that the birth is near, you may long to get it over with, and start your new life.

> **“** It is important that you allow yourself to express any recurrent emotions, doubts or anxieties that you have, so that you can deal with them and release the tension they create. **”**

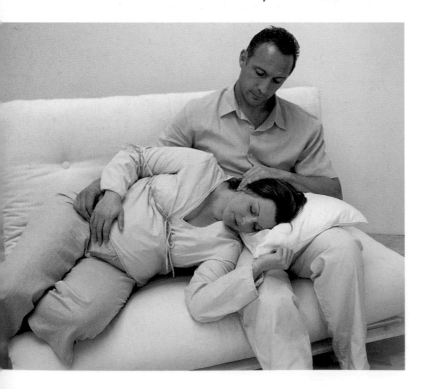

## A LIFE TRANSITION

The strong and fluctuating emotions associated with pregnancy may intensify in the final months, although many women find that they start to feel much calmer as the birth approaches.

Some women feel sad about the loss of freedom having a first baby entails, even if the baby is very much wanted. Many women find themselves worrying about something quite minor – such as where they will put the baby clothes or how they will find time to exercise after the delivery. Almost every pregnant woman feels anxious about the pain of labour and worries that she will not achieve the birth she is expecting.

All these feelings are normal and natural. However, it is important that you allow yourself to express any recurrent emotions, doubts or anxieties that you have, so that you can deal with them and release the tension they create.

Talk to your partner so that he can understand what you are going through and offer you support. This may encourage him to share any ambivalent or difficult emotions that he is experiencing. If you are on your own, talk to a close friend or relative. It can also be invaluable to share your experiences with other pregnant women or with mothers. Your midwife is another good source of support and reassurance.

## YOUR RELATIONSHIP

Pregnancy is bound to affect your relationship. For many couples, a new closeness and tenderness emerges. Your partner may develop a new protectiveness towards you. At the same time, you may become aware of a new feeling of vulnerability and dependency – something that can feel very strange to you both.

The emotional turbulence of pregnancy can put pressure on the relationship, too. Your partner may miss the companionship you used to share and find it difficult to cope with mood swings; you may have unreasonable expectations of how much others can do for you, or feel disappointed that your partner does not seem as interested in your pregnancy as you are.

As with most aspects of pregnancy, it is helpful to cultivate a sense of acceptance and enjoyment about these changes. Continue to spend time alone together and to talk about your feelings.

*Couples often draw closer in the later stages of pregnancy, and men commonly feel a new sense of protectiveness towards their partner.*

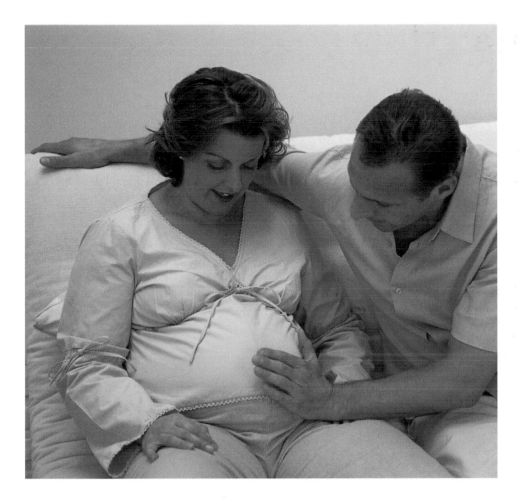

*Talking to the baby regularly will help him or her to become familiar with the voices of both parents. You may even feel your baby respond with a little kick when you start speaking.*

Physical closeness is also important. Massage can be a wonderfully sensuous way of retaining intimacy. Of course, making love will help you to explore any new feelings towards each other. Pregnant women often worry that their partner no longer finds them attractive, particularly in the later stages of pregnancy. However, you may find that your partner enjoys your new curves and voluptuousness. Some couples find that the tenderness pregnancy can evoke – as well as the need to experiment with new positions – brings a new element to their love-making. Other couples find it hard to contemplate the idea of having sex late in pregnancy.

There are no rights and wrongs here – and it is best to do what you feel most comfortable with. But if you both want to make love, sex can usually continue until the waters have broken, as long as the pregnancy is progressing normally. Check with your midwife or doctor if you are not sure.

## THE FATHER-TO-BE

The third trimester can be an exciting time for fathers. The baby is becoming more and more visible and active, and may respond at the sound of the father's voice.

However, late pregnancy also has its challenges. Inevitably the attention is on the pregnant women and some men can feel rather isolated and redundant. This is a false impression: the woman needs their support and love more than anyone else's.

New fathers do have a lot to contend with – and this is something that is rarely recognized. If they are to be the main breadwinners for a while, they may well worry about how they will cope with the extra burden. In addition, men often grow nervous about how the baby will affect their lives. They might find themselves wondering if they will ever again be able to go out for a quiet drink once the baby has arrived.

Becoming a parent is a huge event and it is natural for fathers to have anxieties. Expressing these fears will make them seem more manageable, and will help fathers to support their partners.

As well as talking to their partners, father could try seeking out other fathers. It can really help to talk to someone who has been in the same situation. Another man is likely to have a similar perspective and may have dealt with the same feelings.

### COUNSELLING
You may want to consider seeking help from a counsellor if your emotions become overwhelming and you feel that you cannot cope alone.

# Feel-good treats and therapies

Many women revel in the changes that late pregnancy brings, enjoying their new voluptuousness. However, others dislike becoming so much larger and heavier, particularly if their weight has been an issue before conceiving.

Pregnancy can certainly be a challenge to your self-image, and many women find it hard to cope with stretch marks, varicose veins and other visible ailments. However, it is important to develop a sense of acceptance and appreciation of your body in these last months. This will not only help you to enjoy pregnancy, but it will enhance your general feeling of well-being.

Touch is one of the best ways to maintain a sense of connection with your physical self. Try regular self-massage or enjoy massage with your partner. Gentle exercise, particularly walking, swimming and yoga will help you to feel good. Above all – treat yourself. Incorporating indulgent moments into every day and looking after yourself physically will help you to embrace your growing body. This, in turn, will help you to enjoy the journey towards motherhood.

### LOOK GOOD, FEEL GOOD

Making an effort to look good can often improve the way you feel. Try these quick fixes.

- Get your hair cut. Having a good haircut is one of the quickest ways to make yourself feel attractive. This is probably not the time to go for a radical style – choose something that you know suits you.
- Have a manicure. Even if you don't usually worry about how your hands look, late pregnancy can be a great time to spoil yourself.
- Buy something new to wear. By now, you are probably heartily sick of all the maternity clothes you

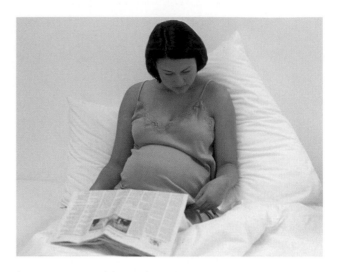

*Late pregnancy is one time when you can enjoy being lazy without feeling guilty – after all, your baby needs you to rest. Go to bed for the afternoon with a glossy magazine or paper, and indulge yourself.*

have bought so far. Women often feel guilty about spending money on clothes they are going to wear for only a few months, with the result that they make do with two or three outfits throughout their pregnancy. However, one new outfit can lift your self-esteem and help you to feel happy about the way you look.
- Wear clothes in natural fabrics, which are softer and more comfortable than manmade materials. Colour therapists often recommend green or blue as good colours to wear during pregnancy because they have a calming effect. Yellow can also be a good choice since it can lift the spirits. But, most importantly, choose clothes in a colour that you feel good in.

### PAMPER YOURSELF

Late pregnancy is a good time to indulge yourself. Set some time aside to do things that you really enjoy – such as meeting a friend for a long catching-up session, reading a novel, going for a walk in the park, or one of the following:
- Buy yourself a large bunch of flowers and put them somewhere you will see them often.
- Book a meal in a favourite restaurant for you and your partner. Enjoy spending a romantic evening together as a couple. Book the table for the earlier part of the evening so that you can still get a good night's rest.

*Enjoy small extravagances, such as buying yourself a bouquet of beautiful fresh flowers.*

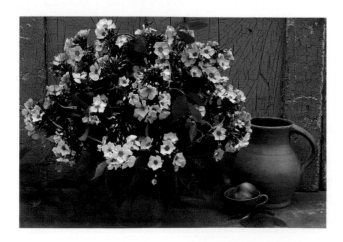

- Spend an afternoon or a whole day in bed. Forget about chores, preparing for the baby or working. Enjoy getting up late, reading the papers or a book or just dozing for a day.
- Go to the cinema, theatre, opera or ballet. It will be much more difficult to organize nights out once the baby is born, so make the most of these last weeks. Go to an afternoon or an early-evening show if you usually feel tired later in the evening.

## NATURAL THERAPIES

A treatment with a qualified complementary therapist can boost your energy and help to relieve some of the discomforts of late pregnancy. The following can also be deeply pleasurable to receive:

- **Reflexology** Few things are more relaxing than a foot treatment. Find a professional reflexologist who specializes in treating pregnant women – some points can stimulate contractions of the uterus.
- **Reiki** You can receive reiki sitting up and fully clothed. It is gentle, soothing and non-invasive. The practitioner places his or her hands on or just above different areas of your body. You may feel a warm or tingling sensation as healing energy flows through the practitioner's hands to wherever it is needed.
- **Shiatsu** This Japanese massage is given on the floor, and you remain clothed. It can be deeply relaxing,

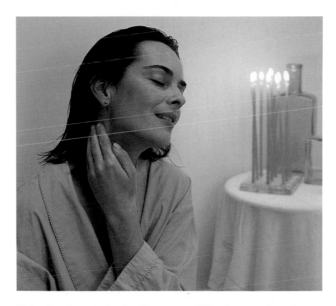

*Take the time to look after yourself in the evening: have a warm bath, wrap yourself in a robe and apply a mask or deep moisturizer to your face.*

and acupressure points may be used to relieve common symptoms such as fatigue. See a practitioner who is experienced with pregnancy. Tell them if you have any varicose veins, as direct pressure should not be applied to them. Abdominal work and heavy pressure on the legs should also be avoided.

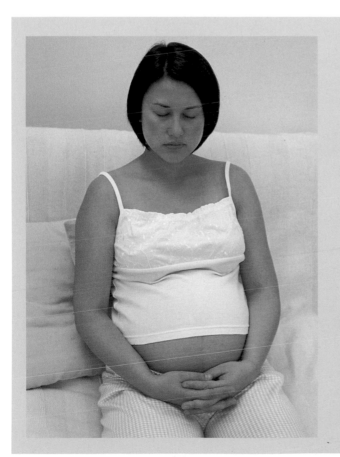

## POSITIVE THINKING

If you are finding it hard to embrace the physical changes of pregnancy, try doing this exercise for five or ten minutes. It will work best if you do it daily.

Sit in a comfortable position, ideally with your back straight. If you have back problems or are feeling tired, prop yourself up against a pile of cushions. Take a few deep breaths, allowing your body to release any tension.

Silently focus on an affirmative phrase about the physical changes you are experiencing. Your affirmation should be a short, positive phrase in the present tense. Make up your own or try one of the following:

I am growing more and more beautiful every day.
I welcome and embrace the changes in my body.

Continue to breathe deeply as you repeat the affirmation over and over. Don't worry if you don't feel what you are saying is true – just keep on silently repeating yourself. Eventually, the message will sink in.

When you are ready to finish, bring your attention back to your breathing. Now, slowly open your eyes. Remain sitting quietly for a minute before you get up.

*Positive affirmations can shift negative feelings about yourself and help you to enjoy your pregnancy more.*

# Perineal and breast massage

Massage of the perineum and breasts is both pleasant and beneficial during the last trimester. Regular massage of the perineum, the area between the vagina and rectum, may help to reduce the chance of tearing during the birth. Massaging your breasts will help to prepare them for breastfeeding. You need not use oil to massage these areas, although you may well find it easier to do so. Use pure, plain oils such as wheatgerm, olive or almond oils, avoiding any that are contraindicated during pregnancy. If you want to use any oils not mentioned below, then consult an aromatherapist first.

### PERINEAL MASSAGE

The perineum has to be strong to support the contents of the abdomen, especially as your baby grows heavier. At the same time, however, the perineum will also have to yield and stretch in order to let your baby pass down the birth canal. Nature provides for this change in texture by releasing "loosening" hormones that soften the ligaments. You can also help to improve elasticity in this area by self-massage. Massaging gently can greatly increase the comfort and ease with which you give birth, and possibly prevent a tear or the need for a surgical cut (episiotomy).

It is truly amazing just how quickly the normally tight tissues in the perineum and vagina will stretch with regular massage. The more that you are able to pre-stretch these tissues before the birth, the better you will return to your original shape after it.

During the last weeks of pregnancy (starting around 36 weeks), massage the perineal area once a day for around five or ten minutes, always doing so with great care and sensitivity. Ideally, perform the massage after soaking in a warm (not hot) bath, to soften the area, and when your bladder is empty. If using oil, wheatgerm is a good choice, and aromatherapists recommend adding a few drops of lavender to the oil.

### HOW TO MASSAGE THE PERINEUM

When you start practising perineal massage, use two fingers, oiled if you wish. Insert the two fingers into your vagina up to the first knuckle, progressing to the second

*For massage of the perineal and vaginal areas, make sure you are in a relaxed and comfortable position. Lying on your side against a bed or beanbag is a good position, as is squatting or half-kneeling with one leg up.*

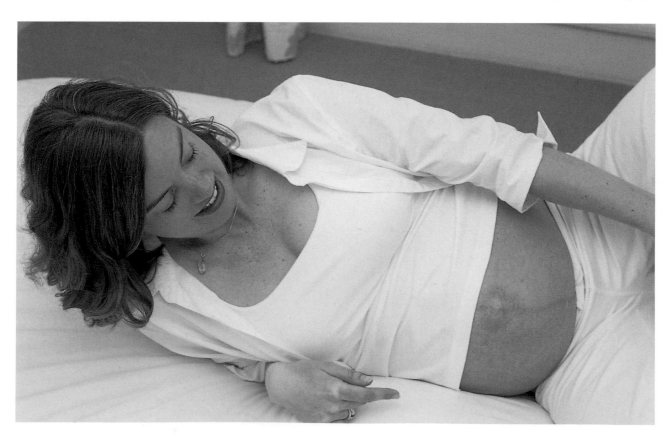

knuckle with practice. You may like to use three or four fingers, and apply a little more pressure, once you are used to the technique. Now use a light touch to explore the layers of tissues along the back wall of your vagina and the skin that separates your vagina and anus. It is this area that will be most stretched during the birth of your baby and is most prone to tearing.

As you press against the back wall of the vagina, against the spine, breathe deeply. You will experience a tingling sensation and will feel the muscles under your fingers as they engage on the breath out. As space is gradually created, move in further and exert a little more pressure, using your breath to help you, but you should never take this kind of massage any further than feels totally comfortable.

You will probably find that nothing much seems to happen at first, but soon your perineal tissue starts to give and then begins to stretch. You will be amazed how much you can stretch it, simply by breathing out into the areas under your fingers.

## MASSAGING THE BREASTS

Up to around 36 weeks, regular massage of the breasts is a wonderful way of bringing a combination of tone, strength and elasticity to the tissues here, in readiness for breastfeeding. Remember to avoid the nipple area. If you decide to use oil then almond oil is a good choice. Calendula cream is also gentle and safe. Like perineal massage, breast massage is best done after a warm and relaxing bath.

To massage the breasts, use your entire hand, with your fingers kept together. With each stroke, start with the heel of your hand and take the stroke through your fingers. Keep the pressure even and smooth; do not jab or press harshly.

In order to understand the technique, you need to imagine the ducts that carry breast milk rather like the spokes of a wheel, radiating out from the central spoke – your nipple. The milk travels down these ducts to the

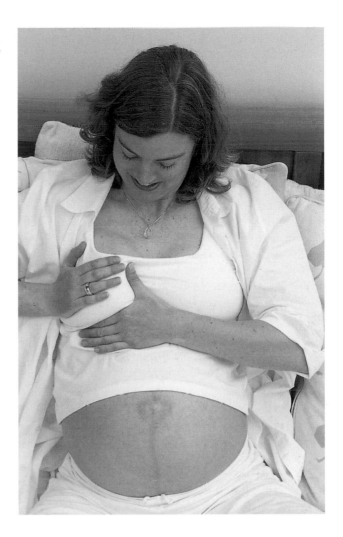

*When massaging the breasts, either massage through clothes or directly on to the skin. As well as massage, you may find that exposing your breasts to the elements from time to time will feel especially pleasant.*

nipple, and your massage should also work from the outside of the breast towards the nipple. Do this slowly around the whole of each breast, working in a clockwise direction. Many pregnancy books compare the breast to a clockface, and recommend starting at 1 o'clock, working from the outside in to the nipple, then repeating this at 2 o'clock and so on.

## MASSAGING OTHER AREAS

While you are in a relaxed mood, with suitable oils at the ready, it is a good idea to extend your massage to other areas of the body. A facial massage is always enjoyable (see page 59) and you could also try gentle massage of the abdomen, in order to help prevent stretch marks. During the latter weeks of pregnancy, massage down the sides of your belly. Work from the ribs to your navel, with both hands and using circular strokes, and continue down over your hips and thighs. Using plenty of oil feels especially pleasant when massaging the abdomen.

### SAFETY POINTS

Take great care with perineal or vaginal massage, and never deliberately stretch out or pull these very delicate tissues.

Do not perform breast massage after about 36 weeks. When massaging the breasts, always proceed gently and avoid massaging the nipples themselves. However, a very gentle tweaking of the nipples can be appropriate once your due date has arrived. This tweaking is said to stimulate production of the hormone oxytocin and so may help to bring on labour.

# Yoga for the third trimester

You will find that your baby is sensitive to your moods, shares your enjoyment and joins in with many of your activities. So the more that you dance around and stretch, and open and tone your body, the better he or she will like it. Your centre of gravity lies deep within your pelvis. The opening up of your hips and pelvic area, plus all the activity, will encourage your baby to find the very best position to be in as birth approaches. Putting aside time each day for a few minutes of energetic yoga dance, followed by a perineal stretch, is a great way to prepare for labour with your baby and it will also help release tension. Don't forget that all these rotating, twisting and opening movements of the hips should be done with knees bent. Keep breathing deeply all the time.

## Knee circles

This is a balancing exercise that shakes out your hips and legs as you get into a knee-swinging stride. It is a loosening and strengthening movement, which helps to boost the circulation and is also good for lifting your mood. If you feel wary about trusting your balance, try placing one hand against a wall for support. Keep your arms, shoulders and neck relaxed. The raised leg is also kept as loose as possible throughout, and the knee circles should be done smoothly and lightly. Before you start, stand erect and breathe deeply for a few moments.

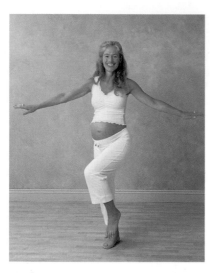

**1** Raise your left leg, bending the knee. Stand on your right leg, with your arms spread out to the sides to help your balance, and your spine erect. Now swing your left knee up in front of you as high as is comfortable.

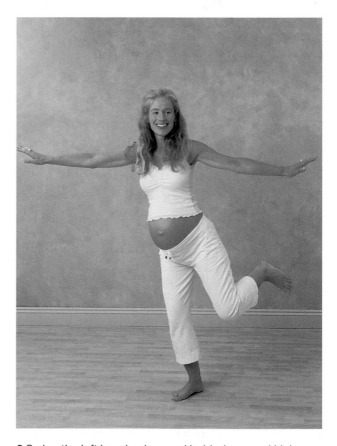

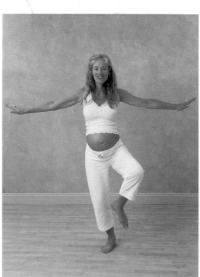

**2** Bring your left knee to the side to open your left hip and so make more room in the abdomen and pelvis.

**3** Swing the left leg slowly round behind you and kick back with your left foot. Finally, swing your knee forward, then straighten your left leg and place your left foot firmly on the floor. Repeat the exercise with the right knee.

## Pushing the sky

In this empowering pose, you are pushing your palms up into the sky. The aim is to lift and strengthen your upper body, and to make space in your lower body as you flex your thigh muscles. Use your diaphragm and breathe deeply, so that you involve all your abdominal muscles in the action.

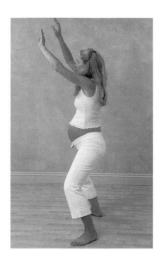

**1** Stand with feet wide and toes pointing outwards so that you can bend your knees deeply and hold this position comfortably. Keeping the spine erect and coccyx tucked in, raise your arms. Push up further with first one palm and then the other. Turn your palm upwards if you can. Feel a lengthening stretch up through each side of your body in turn.

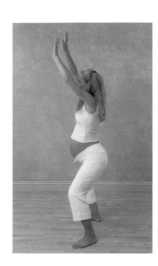

**2** Keep your arms raised directly over your head. Push both hands upwards while bending the knees further and dropping into a semi-squat. Do this on an outbreath, feeling a lengthening stretch through your middle as you do so.

## Standing twist

This is a good position for easing tension in the neck and shoulders, and it also acts as a counter-pose to the strong sideways stretch of the Knee circles. Breathe deeply and twist through the whole torso.

## Seated perineal stretch

A low stool and several cushions are useful props for this gentle perineal stretch, which is good preparation for the birth. Place one cushion on the stool and the others under your dropped knee as required in Step 2. The breath is very important when you are stretching the yogic way – otherwise nothing happens, or you simply stretch a little in the groin area. Remember to move gently and slowly.

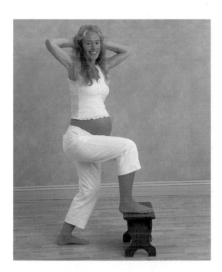

Place your right foot on a low stool, thigh parallel to the floor. Raise your arms and open the elbows to expand the chest. Place your palms behind your head, neck erect. Breathe in. As you breathe out, turn the head and shoulders to the right. Let your chest follow, but keep your lower body steady. Come back to the centre, change legs and repeat on the left.

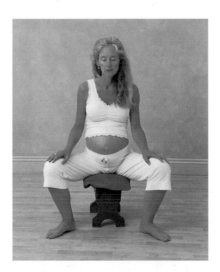

**1** Place a cushion on a low stool and sit astride it, with your knees wide and feet firmly planted on the floor. Stretch up through your spine by pressing the palms of your hands against your spread thighs. Breathe normally but evenly as you do this.

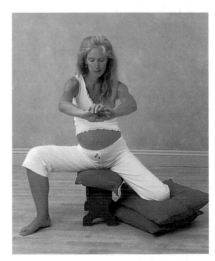

**2** Press into your right foot and drop the left knee back and down on to two firm cushions. This is a good stretch for the perineum and the left groin. Clasp your hands. Inhale as you push the palms away, pressing further into your right foot. Push out further as you exhale and lift through the spine as you inhale. Do this several times. Change legs and repeat.

# Hip-openers in water

Here are some good yoga exercises to do in the swimming pool. The buoyant water supports your weight, making it much easier to stretch and move around. In these exercises one leg is raised to rotate and open the hip, involving all the lower back muscles on that side as well as the pelvic muscles. They both prevent and relieve lower backache, particularly sciatica or inflammation. Start with the small knee circles, then proceed to the wider hip circles. Do them very slowly, with your leg moving as much water as possible.

## Knee circles

For this exercise, face the wall and hold on to the bar or edge of the pool, or face the pool and rest your arms on a woggle (long float) in front of you. The same exercise can be done facing the pool and supporting yourself on the bar or edge from behind, or on a woggle under your arms and behind your back. While facing the wall, the main stretch is in the lower back; facing the pool a greater emphasis is placed on opening the pelvis.

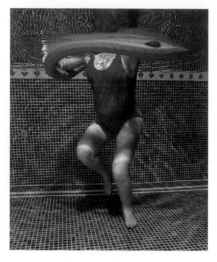 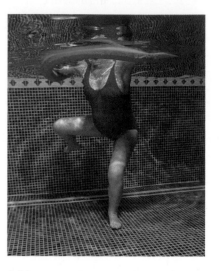

**1** Start in a standing position. Bend the knee of your standing leg slightly. Lift your other leg up from the pool floor, bending your knee as you do so. Keep your upper body relaxed.

**2** Move your knee to make small smooth circles in the water. Keep your whole body relaxed and feel the resistance of the water. Change legs and repeat the exercise.

## Hip circles

Start in a standing position, facing the wall and holding on to the bar or the edge of the pool, or resting your arms on a woggle in front of you. Keep your standing leg a little more bent than for the knee circles, to allow for a wider opening of your other leg as you engage your hip in the rotating movement.

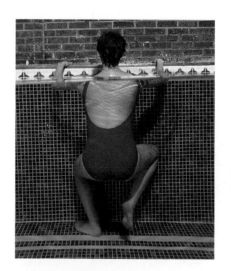 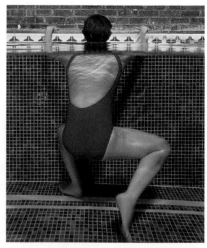

**1** Lift one leg, bending the knee. Slowly circle the hip and knee, feeling the resistance of the water as you do so. Make small circles at first.

**2** Gradually increase the size of the circles by pushing your raised knee back. Exhale each time you open out the knee. Repeat on the other side.

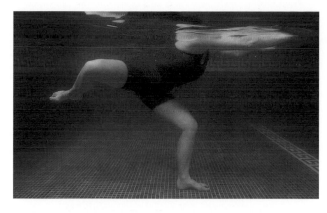

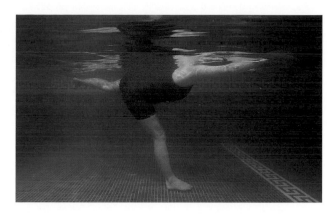

**3** Move away from the side of the pool. Make larger circles, stretching the leg out to the side, then bending it again to come back to the centre. Do this a few times. Breathe deeply, using your abdominal muscles.

**4** Now extend your raised leg back behind you before bringing it back. As you become fitter, extend your leg higher towards the surface of the water, straightening your standing leg.

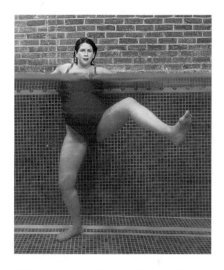

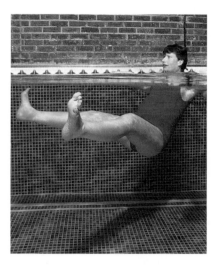

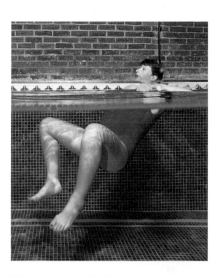

**5** Move so your back is facing the side of the pool or place a woggle under your arms for support. Make circles with your leg, opening the hips wide on each side while keeping your back straight.

**6** Supporting your extended arms on the bar, pool edge or a woggle, work both your hips at the same time, using a wide backstroke movement with your legs.

**7** Now stretch the legs out in front of you, inhaling as you do so. Bend the legs in as you exhale. Keep the upper part of your body as relaxed as possible.

**8** Complete the routine by bringing both legs together and making a rotating movement. Do small circles at first, then gradually increase the size of the circle, breathing deeply all the time. With practice, your circling will start to become smoother and more regular.

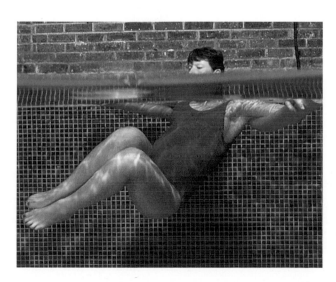

# Antenatal care

The three cornerstones of antenatal care at this stage of your pregnancy are: attending antenatal checks; going to antenatal classes; and looking after your general health.

## ANTENATAL CHECKS

Most women attend their antenatal clinic every month until about the 28th week, fortnightly until about week 36 and then weekly until the birth. During your antenatal visits, the following routine checks will be carried out:

- Weight.
- Blood pressure, to detect pre-eclampsia.
- Urine, to detect signs of pre-eclampsia and diabetes.
- The baby's heartbeat.
- The size of your abdomen, in order to monitor the baby's continuing growth.
- Your hands and legs for any sign of swelling, which could indicate pre-eclampsia.

### Your blood pressure

Pregnancy brings about enormous changes in blood volume and pressure, partly because your heart is beating much faster and more frequently than usual and partly because of hormonal changes in the blood vessels. Your blood pressure will usually return to normal within a few days of the birth.

High blood pressure early in pregnancy can indicate a number of conditions, including kidney disease and diabetes. In later pregnancy, raised blood pressure alone does not usually signify problems, but high blood pressure combined with swelling of the ankles or feet, pronounced weight gain and the appearance of protein in the urine are signs of pre-eclampsia, which develops in about one in every 20 pregnancies.

### What is pre-eclampsia?

Pre-eclampsia is not yet fully understood, but it is believed to be due to abnormalities of hormone secretion, kidney secretion, or the production of abnormal substances by the placenta. Mild pre-eclampsia is usually simple to treat: rest may be all that is needed. Left untreated, it can progress to eclampsia, which is a dangerous complication of pregnancy.

An eclamptic fit dramatically reduces the oxygen supply to the unborn baby, and can also be life-threatening to the mother. If a fit occurs, the baby will be delivered immediately either by induction or by emergency Caesarean. You may not notice any symptoms if you have pre-eclampsia, which is one reason why

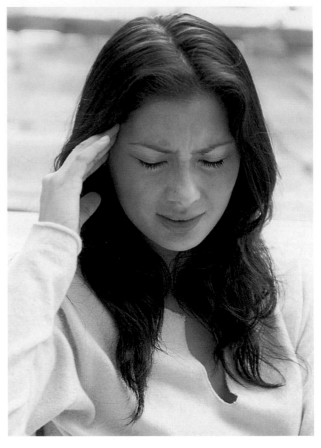

*A severe headache accompanied by blurred vision or flashing lights could be a sign of pre-eclampsia.*

antenatal checks are so vital. The symptoms of this condition can include:

- Severe headache.
- Visual disturbances such as flashing lights or blurring.
- Vomiting.
- Severe pain in the upper abdomen.
- Feet, ankles or hands swelling up suddenly.

Seek immediate medical advice if you develop any of the symptoms listed above during your pregnancy; you must call an ambulance if any of them are severe.

❝ If you or your partner are in any doubt about an aspect of your health, your baby's health or your antenatal health care, seek professional advice. ❞

### The 32-week scan

You will probably have had a scan around week 20 of your pregnancy. If you are receiving specialist antenatal care because of an identified risk factor in your pregnancy, you may have another scan at about 32 weeks. This allows the accurate measurement of the baby's head and abdomen. The information obtained from the scan at this stage of development is more precise than that obtained from a physical examination.

## LOOKING AFTER YOUR HEALTH

During the third trimester, you should still be eating healthily every day, taking some exercise and avoiding smoky atmospheres and alcohol. It is especially important at this stage that you make every effort to keep stress at bay and make sure that you get plenty of relaxation, rest and sleep each day. This will stand you in good stead not only for the birth itself, but also for dealing with your newborn baby once he or she arrives.

If you or your partner are in any doubt about an aspect of your health, your baby's health or your antenatal health care, never hesitate to seek professional advice. The family doctor, your midwife, your hospital, and your antenatal class teacher are there to answer any questions that you may have.

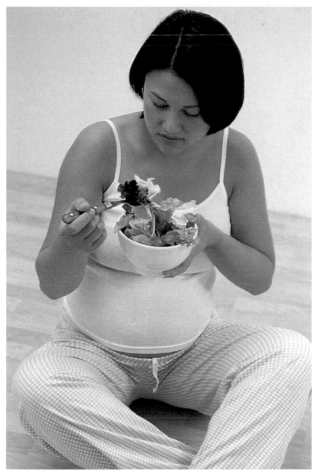

*Look after yourself and your baby by continuing with a healthy lifestyle – the food you eat and the amount of exercise and relaxation you get are all important.*

### WHEN THE BABY COMES EARLY

A pre-term baby is one that arrives or has to be delivered for medical reasons up to three weeks before the estimated date of delivery. A premature baby is one that has arrived more than three weeks early. He or she has an increased chance of respiratory problems in the first few days, and may need special care. Drugs can be given to activate the baby's lungs artificially to speed them towards maturity. These work only if administered early in the third trimester (about weeks 29–33), and are given only if doctors are about to deliver the baby. Once the baby is born, he or she can be put on a ventilator to assist with breathing. The baby also needs to be kept very warm while he or she builds up the fat reserves that would normally have built up by delivery.

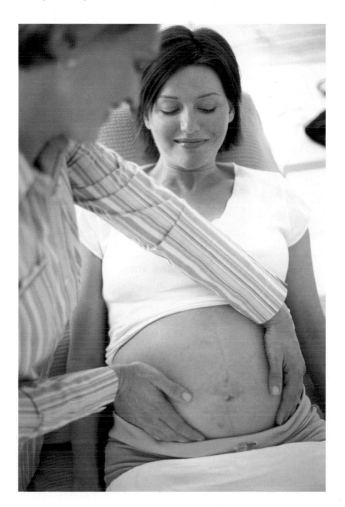

*During each antenatal visit, the midwife will feel your abdomen to check the increase in the size of your uterus, and therefore the growth of your baby.*

# Antenatal classes

The various kinds of antenatal classes are quite distinct from antenatal care, which you receive in an antenatal clinic. While the clinics concentrate mainly on your health and that of your baby, antenatal classes cover the practical and emotional aspects of pregnancy and labour. Classes usually cover a wide range of topics, from sex during pregnancy to pain relief at the birth.

Many women find antenatal classes helpful. You are not only given valuable information, but the classes also provide an opportunity for you to ask any questions that you may have and to swap experiences with other women at the same stage of pregnancy as you. Women often forge friendships at antenatal classes that continue long after the birth of their babies. These can be a good source of support during the first months of motherhood.

Antenatal classes are known by various names: for example, parentcraft, childbirth education classes or preparation for parenthood. Active birth classes – which encourage the use of yoga – may also be available. Classes are run by different organizations, such as the health authority, charities and independent teachers. Your doctor or midwife will tell you about the different classes on offer, and you can choose a system that suits you.

The classes usually run weekly for five to six weeks, perhaps eight weeks, and you attend them during the last couple of months of pregnancy. Most classes actively encourage male partners to come along, and offer specific advice for them. However, you can also go on your own or take a friend or relative along with you.

*Antenatal classes help you understand exactly what happens during pregnancy and childbirth. Here a teacher uses models of a baby and a pelvis to demonstrate the breech (feet or buttocks first) position.*

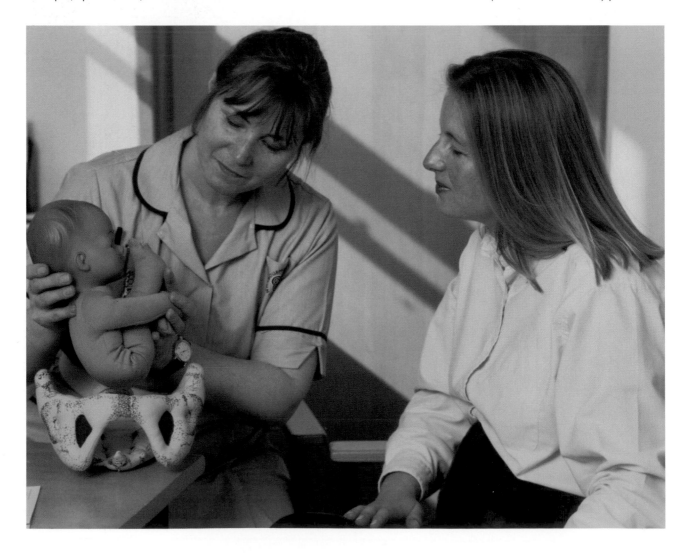

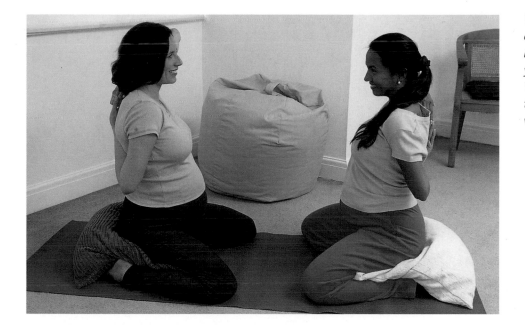

*You will learn simple exercises to relieve backache and to prepare your body for the birth. You can then practise these regularly at home with a friend.*

## WHAT ANTENATAL CLASSES COVER

Antenatal classes will always include an opportunity for you and your partner to ask any questions that you may have. The classes will usually also cover set topics each week, which will include all or most of the following:

### Pregnancy

- Diet, health and fitness in pregnancy.
- Caring for your teeth and gums.
- Bathing in pregnancy.
- Posture and back problems.
- Maternity clothing.
- Relationships and sex during pregnancy.
- Talks for partners covering pregnancy, the birth and fatherhood.
- How the baby grows – the developmental milestones of the unborn baby.
- Coping with common discomforts such as piles, constipation and back pain.
- Exercises, including pelvic floor exercises, to help you prepare for the birth and to prevent problems such as stress incontinence.

### The birth

- Breathing exercises for labour. In antenatal classes, you are taught how to change your breathing deliberately during labour, adjusting to the changing characteristics of the contractions. This can help you to manage your labour and cope better with the pain. Synchronizing the breathing with the signals that are received from the uterus demands total concentration and it is important to practise the techniques regularly beforehand.

Many classes will include special advice for your partner or a friend, who will then be able to assist you and provide support in labour.

- A visit to the maternity ward and labour ward. This will help you to understand the technology of birth: medical terms will be explained and you'll have an opportunity to see some of the equipment. You'll also get a chance to see what options are available in your particular unit (for example, water births), and to become familiar with the wards and labour suite.
- What you will need for a home birth.
- How to recognize the signs of labour.
- What happens during labour.
- Options for pain relief during labour.
- Breech births.
- Medical intervention, such as induction, Caesarean section and assisted deliveries.

### After the birth

- Breast and bottle-feeding.
- Caring for the nipples when breastfeeding; coping with other associated problems, such as mastitis.
- What you will need after the birth for yourself – maternity bras and other clothing.
- What you will need for the baby – equipment and clothing.
- Basic baby-care skills – including how to change a nappy and how to bath a baby.
- How to recognize postnatal depression.
- Advice on contraception after delivery, because you can become pregnant quite quickly after the arrival of your baby. It is best to delay conceiving again for at least nine months after the birth.

# Checklist of common problems

Your baby almost doubles in size during the third trimester, and your body has to stretch and grow to accommodate it. Not surprisingly, most women feel heavy and uncomfortable during this stage of pregnancy.

It can be difficult to find a comfortable sleeping position, so you may feel very tired. You may also suffer from breathlessness, since the expanding uterus presses up against the lungs, or from circulation problems, such as swollen ankles.

Make sure that you get plenty of rest during the day, especially if you are sleeping badly at night, and put your feet up regularly. If you are suffering from other minor ailments, complementary therapies can often help to relieve them. However, always check the relevant safety advice in Chapter Six, and talk to your midwife or doctor before using any remedy.

You should report any symptoms you are experiencing to your midwife during your antenatal visits. See your doctor beforehand if symptoms are severe, persistent or concern you in any way.

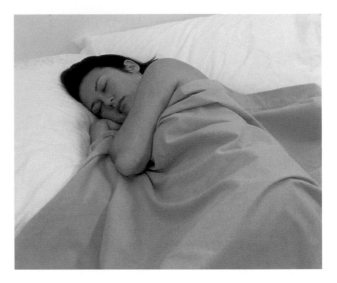

*Sleep is an excellent restorative. Make sure you get as much as possible in these last weeks of pregnancy. You need to be well rested for the labour.*

**Cramp** Leg cramps often occur in late pregnancy. They may be caused by deficiencies of calcium and magnesium, so try eating more dairy products, sardines and green leafy vegetables (for calcium) and plenty of nuts and seeds (for magnesium). Vitamin B2, which is found in yogurt, lean meat and fortified breakfast cereals, may help. You should make sure that you drink plenty of water and take regular exercise. If you do get cramp, rub your calf briskly. Try flexing your foot at the same time so that the toes point upwards.

**Stress incontinence** Leaking urine can be an embarrassing problem, but it is one that many pregnant women experience. It is usually caused by weakness of the pelvic floor, which supports the neck of the bladder. To prevent stress incontinence, practise pelvic floor exercises several times a day: tighten the ring of muscles around your vagina and anus, as though you were stopping yourself from urinating mid-flow. Hold for a count of five, then release. Repeat five times or more.

You are most likely to leak urine when you are lifting, laughing, coughing or sneezing, so pull up the pelvic floor whenever you are about to do so. Regular exercise and yoga can also help to strengthen the pelvic floor.

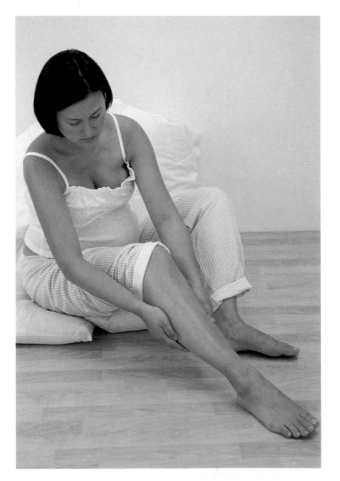

*If you get cramp in the calf, rub briskly, then massage using a squeezing action. Make sure you get some gentle exercise – such as a half-hour walk – each day.*

**Backache**  Almost all pregnant women suffer from backache in the third trimester, and often earlier, too. The growing weight of the baby in your uterus alters your centre of gravity, and you may sit or stand awkwardly to compensate. An Alexander technique teacher can help you to adjust your posture, and chiropractic and osteopathy can also be very beneficial. Regularly practising yoga and Pilates often helps; ask your teacher to recommend specific exercises to do at home. A gentle massage should help to relieve discomfort. Chiropractic and osteopathy are also useful.

**Pubic joint pain**  The pubic joint (symphysis pubis) softens in preparation for childbirth, which places strain on the spine and pelvis. This can cause pain in the pubic area, and sometimes in the lower back and groin as well. Tell your doctor if you are affected; he or she may refer you to a physiotherapist to be fitted with a support belt. Otherwise regular chiropractic or osteopathy sessions can be very helpful. Other therapies that may be useful include acupuncture, reiki, reflexology and the Alexander technique.

**Shortness of breath**  As your uterus expands, it presses against your lungs, which can cause breathlessness or exacerbate respiratory problems such as asthma. Practising abdominal breathing will help to improve your breath control, as will yoga, Pilates and the Alexander technique. If the problem gets worse when you lie down, use pillows to prop yourself up. If you suffer from asthma, try eating more oily fish; fish oils seem to protect against attacks. Homeopathy, aromatherapy, acupuncture, reflexology and reiki may help with both asthma and shortness of breath.

**Indigestion and heartburn**  These problems can get worse in the third trimester, when the growing uterus presses on the stomach. Eating little, often and slowly is the simplest way to prevent them, and you should avoid eating spicy foods. Sipping a cup of lemonbalm or meadowsweet tea after meals may help. If you suffer from heartburn, make sure that you do not bend or lie down for at least an hour after eating.

**Itchy skin**  Hormonal changes during pregnancy can lead to skin problems, particularly during the third trimester. If you have dry, itchy skin, try eating more oily fish, nuts and seeds. Moisturizing your skin with an evening primrose lotion can help, or you may like to use essential oil of lavender or chamomile well-diluted in a carrier cream or base oil. Herbal medicine or homeopathy may also be useful – a homeopath may prescribe sulphur or kali arsenicum. See your doctor if the itching becomes severe.

**Water retention**  Pregnant women often experience mild swelling (oedema) of the ankles, especially during the third trimester. If you have swollen ankles, rest with your feet up for at least 15 minutes twice a day. Regular leg massage – working up the leg – and drinking dandelion tea can be useful. You may also find acupuncture helpful. If you have severe swelling and a headache, see your doctor at once.

**High blood pressure**  Your blood pressure will be checked at every antenatal visit; high blood pressure accompanied by fluid retention and protein in the urine indicates pre-eclampsia. This condition can affect your pregnancy so it is important that you follow any advice given by your doctor. You can help to maintain a healthy blood pressure by taking regular exercise and eating a nutritious diet that includes oily fish and plenty of raw fruits and vegetables; you should also follow a low-salt diet. Reducing stress and practising relaxation techniques, meditation, yoga or t'ai chi is often helpful. You may also like to try herbal medicine, aromatherapy, colour therapy, reiki or reflexology.

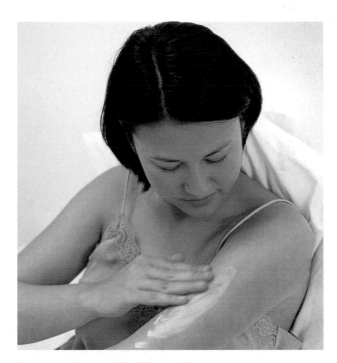

*For immediate relief of itchy skin, use a cream containing evening primrose oil. Increasing the amount of oily fish that you eat should also help.*

**WHEN TO CALL A DOCTOR**
If you experience sudden or severe symptoms, you should contact your doctor or the emergency services without delay. See page 75 for a list of danger signs in pregnancy.

# Common Qs and As

**Q: If I have a row with my partner or my mother, will my baby be affected or harmed by that? Will he or she know?**

**A:** Your baby certainly won't 'know' that you are having an argument in any real sense of the word. He or she will have no means of placing what is said in a meaningful context and assessing it. However, your increasing heart rate and anxiety level will transmit to your baby in some way.

It is best to try to avoid becoming very stressed when you are pregnant, and it will help all of you if you can learn to handle disagreements calmly, through discussion and negotiation and compromise. Once your child is born, he or she will certainly be upset by rows, long before he or she is able to speak.

**Q: I am so huge now, I feel quite otherworldly – as if this is not me – I just want it to be over and see my baby.**

**A:** Many women feel like this towards the last few weeks of their pregnancy, and you are probably experiencing entirely normal feelings. However, it is worth discussing these feelings with your doctor just in case your feelings of depersonalization are associated with depression or acute anxiety. Depression can happen before the birth as well as after it, and it is best treated sooner rather than later.

**Q: I don't know whether I will be able to handle the loss of privacy that giving birth entails. I am a very private person and am worried about the pain, the unknown nature of it all. All my friends seem to have coped better than I think I would.**

**A:** Your question raises a number of issues. First, it would be a good idea to confide your fears and feelings to your family doctor and to the midwife in charge of you so that they can appreciate how you will feel in any given situation. They may well reassure you that many women feel this way. You will also be able to choose not have medical students present for the delivery.

Second, you may well imagine that all your friends have coped better than you think you would. However, this may be supposition on your part. Have you talked to them? Have you asked them if they felt nervous? You may find it helpful to discuss with them how they coped with the pain and loss of privacy.

Third, your own self-esteem may be an issue here. Are you usually confident? Do you often suffer from feelings of lack of confidence or low self-esteem? Experiencing the birth of your baby is without doubt something you can do. It does not matter if you scream or weep – medical staff will have seen other women do the same thing. You should also remember that people will be there to help and comfort you. Rest assured that you will receive the professional assistance and support you need.

Fourth, remember that this is just one day of your life, and you will get through it. Try to see the labour and delivery as a means to an end... seeing your very own gorgeous baby.

**Q**: I am seven months pregnant but I don't feel the emotional bond with my baby that other women talk about. Am I abnormal?

**A**: Not at all. Some women do feel rather detached from their pregnancy, almost as if the baby is growing within them irrespective of the woman herself as a person. Fathers-to-be also often do not bond with their baby until the actual delivery.

However, most parents do feel a surge of love for the baby once he or she is born. The hormones take over and allow you to feel the nurturing, protective love that is normal in parenthood.

If you have any remaining worries after the birth of your baby, be sure to discuss them with your family doctor or your health visitor.

**Q**: Now that I am pregnant, everyone seems to think they can touch my stomach. I really hate being stroked and prodded by strangers but don't know how to stop this happening. What can I do?

**A**: This is an entirely understandable reaction on your part and something expressed by many pregnant women – it is as if people believe that the bump is public property rather than part of your body. Short of staying at home, there is not a lot you can do, except to explain gently that your pregnancy is very personal to you and that you would prefer not to be touched.

**Q**: How will I know when to go to hospital?

**A**: Memorize the warning signs for labour and get your partner or best friend to do the same. They are:
- Breaking of the waters.
- A pinkish show of mucus tinged with blood.
- Contractions becoming regular and pronounced and lasting for some 40 seconds or more. (False labour is characterized by irregular contractions lasting less than 20–30 seconds.)

Ring your midwife if you are in any doubt about whether or not labour has started.

**Q**: What happens if I am caught short – say, if I am on a train or bus – when labour starts? Should I be taking any measures now?

**A**: Labour usually takes some time – and remember that even trains stop. Babies have been delivered in cars, buses, planes and on ships, but obviously one would prefer this not to happen. So, have a fully charged mobile phone with you at all times. From week 38, try to avoid any long journeys away from home and the place where you have chosen to have the delivery. If you are expecting twins, be cautious from week 35 onwards.

**Q**: I have started to worry that my partner may be away when the baby comes – he travels a lot, at short notice, for work – and am feeling panicky about what to do if he is.

**A**: In this situation, you may prefer to have a close friend or relative staying with you, or on stand-by, for the final stages, so make sure you have someone lined up now. If you do not have a friend or relative living close by, talk to your neighbours, who will probably be helpful, and alert your family doctor and midwife to the situation. They may be able to tell you of local back-up services.

# CHAPTER FOUR
# Countdown to birth

**❝** The most important thing to do is to focus on, and prepare yourself for, the labour. **❞**

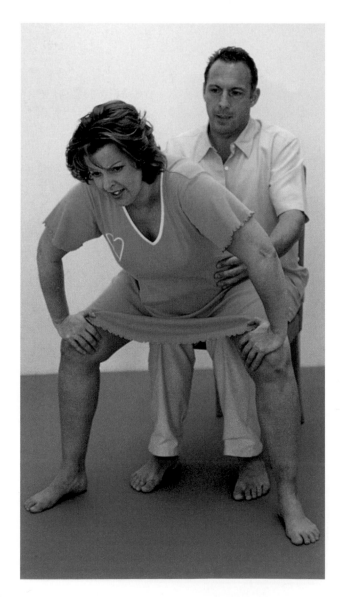

Seeing your new baby for the first time is an entirely magical, joyful and breathtaking moment, an event that you will remember for the rest of your life. Now this moment is just a few weeks away.

As you wait, the most important thing you can do is to focus on, and prepare yourself as much as possible for, the labour and delivery, and for the first weeks of your baby's life. All other considerations – work, socializing, doing the housework – should take second place to this.

You are much larger now and may feel constantly tired. It is more important than ever to focus on rest and relaxation. Avoid becoming overtired because it will be difficult to catch up – once the baby has arrived, your sleep is likely to be repeatedly interrupted. Take a rest in the early afternoon if you can. Drink plenty of water every day in order to expel the toxins from your body and help to reduce general feelings of fatigue.

*Practice makes perfect. Experiment together with different positions for the labour – standing, squatting or kneeling – so you know what to try when the time comes. As you practise, make sure you don't push or exert any downward pressure.*

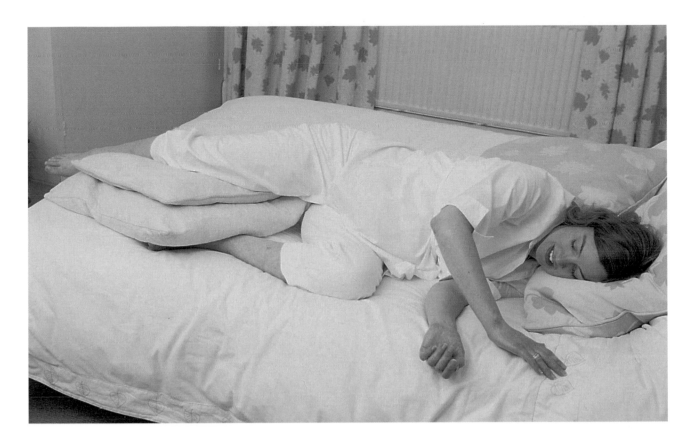

Feed yourself well, regularly and healthily. This will stand you in good stead for the demanding hours of labour and the delivery itself. Gentle activity and antenatal exercises are important in these last few weeks – try to get at least some exercise every day. It is also helpful to prepare mentally for the birth – through breathing, relaxation exercises and visualization, as well as enjoying periods of quiet contemplation each day.

On a practical level, you will probably already have decided on a room or space for your baby. You may be enjoying decorating it and providing for the baby's needs. Creating a welcoming space for your child can be a thrilling experience, and it is a real opportunity for you and your partner to share in the preparations in a practical way.

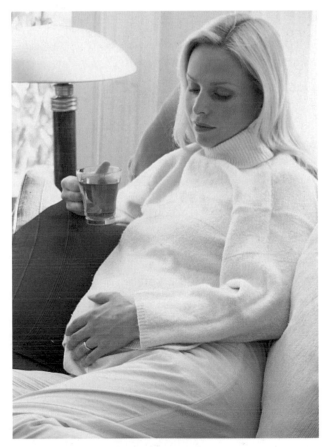

*Top: You may find that this is a particularly comfortable resting position during the very late stages of your pregnancy. Place some padding, such as a pillow or two, under your upper leg in order to relieve pressure on the abdominal blood vessels.*

*Set aside some time each day to sit and relax and be with your unborn child. This can help the mother-child bonding process.*

# Your birth plan

Giving birth is the most personal and intense experience of a woman's life. It is natural that you will want to make it as comfortable and stress-free as possible. Women often have different approaches to giving birth, and midwives and hospitals are now happy to accommodate your preferences where possible.

A birth plan is a note of exactly what you want to happen during and after the birth. Your plan will include details on the type of pain relief you want and who you want to be present. It will also specify whether you want to have your baby at home or in hospital.

Birth plans are highly individual: what suits one woman is not necessarily right for another. It is easy to become overwhelmed by all the options that are open to you, but writing a birth plan can help to clarify your thoughts and preferences. It will also help to highlight any areas where you are unclear about what is possible. You will be able to discuss every aspect of the birth with your midwife. Remember that your midwife is there to help you make the right decisions for you.

Discuss your birth plan with your partner or anyone else you wish to be present at the birth, so that everyone is aware of your wishes. However, bear in mind that circumstances can change. Maintaining a flexible attitude will help you cope if your labour doesn't quite go to plan.

## WHAT IS ON A BIRTH PLAN?

Birth plans vary from country to country and from hospital to hospital, but your plan is likely to include:

- Where you want to give birth.

*Writing a birth plan encourages you to think seriously about all the options available. This can help you to identify what is really important to you – for example, having your aromatherapist present and ensuring that you have access to an epidural if you need one.*

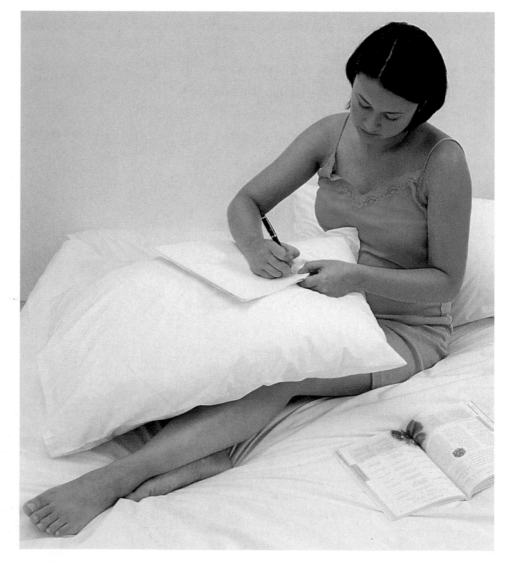

- A note of who you would like to be present (partner, friend, family member, acupuncturist, hypnotherapist).
- What position or positions you hope to adopt for labour and delivery.
- Your feelings about monitoring the baby.
- Your feelings about induction.
- Your feelings about episiotomy.
- Details of what pain relief you want, if any.
- Whether you want the baby put to your chest straight after delivery and before he or she is cleaned up.
- Whether you intend to feed by breast or by bottle.
- How you feel about staying in hospital after the birth.

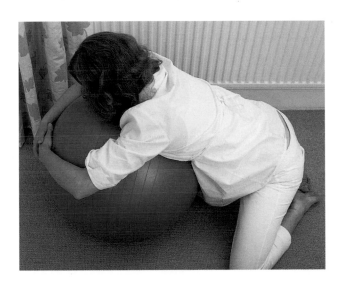

## A FLEXIBLE PLAN

Remember that a birth plan is a list of your preferences rather than an agenda of what is actually going to happen. Labour and delivery can take a different direction in individual cases, acquiring a momentum of their own. Whether or not your birth plan is followed will depend on what happens before, during and after the birth.

Some women prefer not to write a birth plan at all – and it is fine to turn up at the hospital without one. Equally, many women change their mind about certain things. For example, most women would wish to avoid an episiotomy. However, if the baby becomes severely distressed (short of oxygen) and needs to be delivered quickly with forceps, an episiotomy may have to be performed. Equally, some women decide they want to give birth with no pain relief at all. However, it is not possible to predict the degree of pain that may occur nor how easily you will be able to cope with it. In some cases, the woman changes her mind and asks for pain relief.

The birth plan, then, is provisional. It does not commit you to a particular course of action: you may deviate from it if you wish to do so. Medical and nursing staff will also be prepared to deviate from the plan if necessary to preserve your health and the health of the baby.

*Include on the birth plan details of anything that you wish to take into the delivery room – from a birthing ball to soothing chamomile oil or homeopathic tablets.*

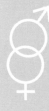

### WHO TO HAVE AT YOUR BIRTH

Most women want someone who they know well to be at the birth – this is usually, but not necessarily, the father. Your birth partner can offer valuable emotional support, act as an advocate with medical staff, and also do simple things to enhance your well-being, such as rub your back or pour you a glass of water when you need one.

Think carefully about who you want to be at the birth, and discuss this with your partner. Most men want to be at the birth of their baby, but a few do not feel able to support their partner in this way. It is usually better to ask a friend or relative to come with you rather than trying to press-gang an unwilling partner.

You may also like to consider asking a complementary therapist to be present for part of your labour. An acupuncturist, for example, may be able to stimulate certain points to ease labour pains, while a homeopath could prescribe remedies for weak contractions or distress.

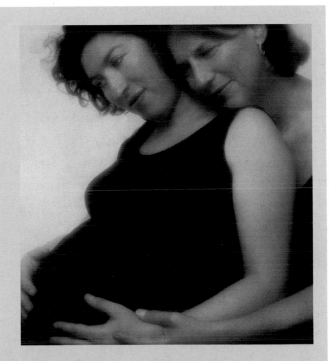

*If you are having the baby on your own or if your partner is unable to be present, take a close friend or relative to support you during the birth.*

# Where to have your baby

The first decision you have to make when planning your birth is where to have your baby – at home or in hospital. Your personal feelings are very important, but you also need to consider any medical issues, as well as your facilities if you want to have a home birth.

You should discuss the issue of where to have your baby with your partner, who may have strong opinions either way. In particular, if you want to have your baby at home, it is important that you have your partner's support.

### HAVING A HOSPITAL BIRTH

The majority of women prefer to give birth in hospital, where there are the medical resources available to deal with any complications that may arise. You will also have access to the complete range of pain relief if you give birth in hospital, and advice and support will be on hand after the birth. The norm is to have a natural (vaginal) delivery, attended by a midwife rather than by a doctor.

However, doctors will be available should you need medical assistance to deliver the baby.

If you deliver normally, you may be encouraged to go home between six and 48 hours later. Women and babies who are unwell after delivery often need to stay longer. The community midwives will continue your care at home for up to ten days, extending to 28 days if necessary.

### HOME BIRTHS

Some women feel more relaxed about the prospect of giving birth in their own environment. One of the advantages of having your baby at home is, of course, that you are the boss. You can watch television in the early stages of labour. You don't have to see anyone that you don't want to see. You can eat when and what you wish. You can have the music and the lighting of your choice. In addition, you can have as many people in the room as you wish.

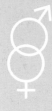

**BEING PREPARED FOR HOSPITAL**
Have a small case or bag packed a few weeks before your estimated date of delivery, so that you are well prepared should the baby come earlier than expected. Have the bag packed at 35 weeks if you are expecting twins or more. You will need most or all of the following:
- Dressing gown.
- Slippers.
- Two nightdresses (which open down the front if you plan to breastfeed).
- Comfortable loose clothes, such as big T-shirts, track pants, skirts.
- Underclothes, including socks and a nursing bra if you want to breastfeed.

- Sanitary towels for after the birth.
- Something to read.
- Sponge bag, containing toothbrush and toothpaste, deodorant, flannel, soap, shampoo, cosmetics, tissues, skin cleanser, moisturizer, cotton wool, scent, wet wipes, nail varnish remover, comb.
- Essential aromatic oils plus electric vaporizer, flower remedies and homeopathic remedies.
- Herbal teas (for example, chamomile or raspberry leaf tea for the labour).
- Facial water spray.
- Address and telephone book.
- Phone card and coins for the telephone (you are often not able to use a mobile phone in a hospital).
- Music and portable stereo.
- Bottled water.
- Snack foods to eat during labour (dried fruit, nuts and raisins, bananas, grapes, carrot sticks, crackers, cheese, yeast extract, cereal bars).
- Sleep suits for your baby.
- Lightweight blanket or shawl.
- Mittens, woolly hat and outdoor suit for the baby.
- A correctly fitted new car seat for your baby to travel home safely.

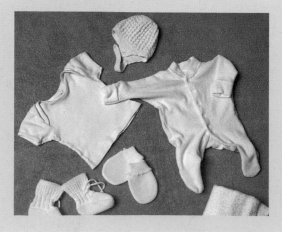

*Don't forget to take one or two outfits to the hospital for your new baby to wear.*

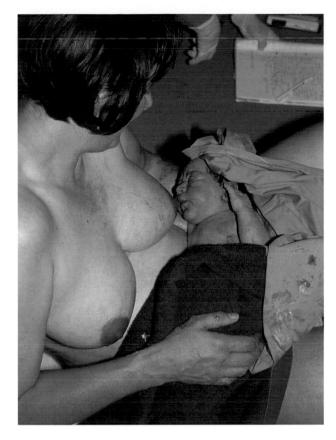

*Giving birth at home gives you greater control over your environment. It also means the first sights, sounds and smells a baby encounters are those of his or her home.*

However, there are disadvantages to home births. The biggest drawback is that you will not have immediate access to specialist medical care if something goes wrong. This is the main reason that many doctors are uncomfortable about the idea of a home birth.

Another consideration may be any other children who live with you. It may prove difficult or distressing for them to hear you in labour, although there is no doubt they will be thrilled when they see the newborn baby. You may wish to arrange for your children to be looked after by a relative or a close friend while you are in labour.

If you give birth at home, it can be more difficult to let go of responsibility for household chores. Make sure that there is someone to look after you who will take over the running of the home. You will not want to answer the telephone or the doorbell within a few hours of giving birth to your baby. There will also have to be someone to clear up and change the bed linen.

## DOCTORS AND HOME BIRTHS

Many doctors understand some women would prefer their baby to be delivered at home. However, they often discourage home births, particularly if there has been any indication that complications may ensue or if you are in a higher-than-average risk category.

If there is a problem during a home birth, valuable time will be lost while arrangements are made for an ambulance to collect the woman and drive her to the hospital. If the complications are serious, this delay could prove life-threatening to either you or your baby.

You may find that your own family doctor will not accept you for antenatal care if you choose to have a home birth. If this is the case, your midwife should be able to put you in touch with another doctor. The delivery will be undertaken by one or two midwives.

### Can you have a home birth?

You have the right to give birth at home. However, if this is your first child or if you are in a high-risk group, a hospital birth will be recommended. The following women are actively discouraged from giving birth at home:

- Women over 35.
- Women expecting twins or more.
- Women expecting their first child.
- Women who had a difficult labour with their first child.
- Women who have had a Caesarean delivery, a stillborn baby, or one who died shortly after birth.
- Anyone who has a serious medical condition that could affect the outcome of the pregnancy and delivery, such as high blood pressure, heart disease, diabetes, significant heart murmur or kidney disease.

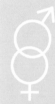

**WHAT YOU WILL NEED AT HOME**
You don't need a lot for a home birth, but the following are essential:

- Adequate heating – the room should be around 20°C (under 70°F).
- Telephone – so that help can be summoned in an emergency.
- Anglepoise lamp so the midwife can see in a dim light.
- Sheets and towels – these should be clean but preferably old so that it doesn't matter if they are stained.
- Clean nightdress for after the birth.
- Sanitary towels.

These items will be helpful:

- Chair and a low stool.
- Several cushions and a large bean bag.
- Natural sponge.
- Mineral water and fruit juice.
- Essential aromatic oils and vaporizer, flower remedies, homeopathic remedies.
- Herbal teas.
- Snack foods to eat during labour (dried fruit, nuts, bananas, grapes, carrot sticks, crackers, cheese, yeast extract, cereal bars).

# Giving birth in water

Whether you are planning to give birth at home or in a hospital, you may wish to opt for a water birth. Midwives have long known that taking a bath can help with relaxation and pain control in early labour. Since the 1980s, an increasing number of women have chosen to spend long periods of their labour in water and to give birth in it. Water births account for approximately one in every 200 births in the UK, and they are also growing in popularity in the United States.

Supporters say that women who spend their labour immersed in warm water benefit in many ways.

- Warm water is naturally soothing and comforting. The pool provides a private space for the labour, which can help the woman to feel more in control.
- Water's buoyancy supports a woman's weight, making it easier for her to relax and change position.
- Water helps to support the pelvic floor and soften the perineum, making women less likely to tear or to require an episiotomy.
- Contractions are less painful because the body is less tense – your body releases pain-killing endorphins when it is in a relaxed state.
- When pain is reduced, women find it easier to concentrate on their breathing, which can help to shorten the labour.
- The father can get in the pool too, making the birth more of a shared experience.

Babies are usually lifted out of the water as soon as they are born, either by the mother, father, midwife or doctor, so that they can breathe. However, the family can usually stay in the water after the birth in order to bond.

## ARE WATER BIRTHS SAFE?

Water births are controversial, and many doctors do not approve of them. However, the *British Medical Journal* conducted a study of all the water births that took place in the UK between 1994 and 1996. It found that the mortality rate for the babies was no greater than that associated with conventional births. There have been no major studies of water births in the United States, and the American College of Obstetrics and Gynecology does not take a stand on the practice.

There has been only limited research into water births, so it is impossible to be entirely sure of the risks. One problem is that it is difficult to maintain the water temperature: if it is too hot, it may cause the baby's heart beat to increase. Another concern is that the baby may be

> **❝** Midwives have long known that taking a bath can help with relaxation and pain control in early labour. **❞**

at risk of drowning. Supporters of water births say this is not possible because the baby does not breathe until he or she comes into contact with the air. However, one report from New Zealand suggested that a few babies have suffered respiratory problems as a result of inhaling water. Many women choose to get out of the water for the actual delivery because of this concern.

If you are considering a water birth, you need to discuss the benefits and risks with your midwife early on. Antenatal classes can be a good source of information, and you may find it helpful to seek out other women who have given birth in this way. Ask your antenatal teacher, search the Internet and look for local support groups.

## CAN I HAVE A WATER BIRTH?

You should be able to have a water birth if your pregnancy has been straightforward and so long as no complications are envisaged. Many hospitals have birthing pools, so in theory water births should be possible in most areas.

In practice, however, the pool may not be available when you need it. For example, it may be being cleaned or in use by another woman. It may be available only if your labour coincides with the shifts of a specific midwife.

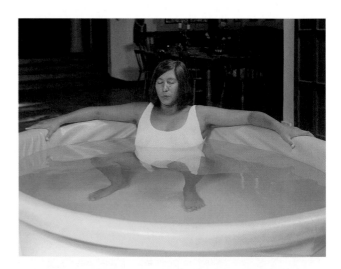

*If you are having a water birth at home, hire the pool a few weeks before your due date. It is a good idea to fill the pool for a trial run beforehand.*

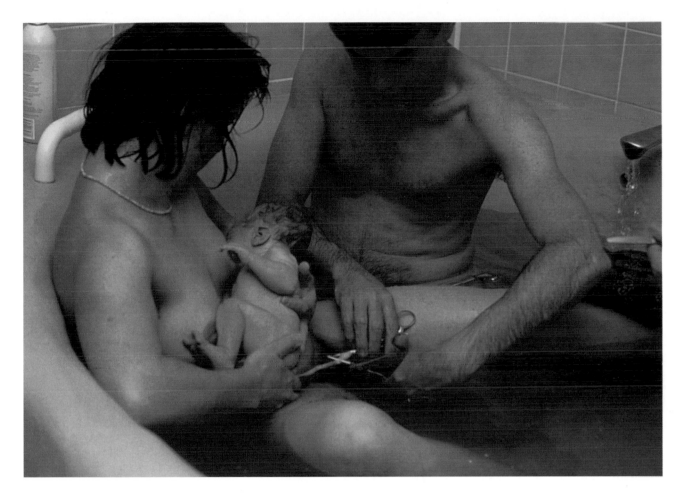

Some hospitals actively discourage women from having a water birth, even if they have the facilities to provide one. Asking these questions should let you see how likely it is that you will be able to have a water birth at your hospital:

- How many women use the birthing pool each year?
- How many women actually give birth in the pool?
- How many midwives are trained to attend water births?
- Will the pool be available when I go into labour?

If you feel that staff are not keen on facilitating a water birth, talk to your midwife. There may be good reasons for this, and it may be that the hospital does not support the practice. If so, you may want to consider having the birth elsewhere. However, make sure you will be assisted by a qualified midwife who is experienced with water births.

### WATER BIRTHS AT HOME
If you are having a home birth, you can hire your own pool. Ask your midwife for details of local companies who rent out pools. Make sure your midwife is happy and confident about facilitating a water birth. If not, ask for a referral to someone who is.

You will need to hire the pool for several weeks, so that you can be sure that you have it when you go into labour. Make sure that your floor can take the weight, and that there is plenty of space around the pool.

*The father may want to get into the birthing pool to share the first moments of his baby's life, or even to cut the umbilical cord, under instruction from the midwife.*

### WHEN WATER BIRTHS ARE UNSUITABLE
Water births are not recommended if the baby is in the breech position; if you are expecting twins; if the baby is more than two weeks early; if you have an infection or other medical condition, or if there is meconium (the baby's first bowel movement) in the amniotic fluid.

It is also important that women do not get into the pool too early in their labour. You should wait until you are at least 5cm (2in) dilated, otherwise the relaxing effects of the water can slow labour down.

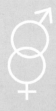

### STAY FLEXIBLE
If you are planning a water birth, remember that labour does not always go to plan. If complications occur, you will need to get out of the pool so that medical assistance can be given. Also, bear in mind that the main aim of a water birth is to facilitate relaxation and well-being: don't turn getting one into a stressful event.

# Preparing for the birth

Many women feel a growing sense of confidence and ease as the due date approaches. However, there can still be moments of anxiety about the birth ahead. You may also have times when you feel very bored – these last few weeks can seem to last forever. Fluctuating emotions are normal in pregnancy. However, it will help you to cope with the birth if you are feeling as emotionally strong as possible. Try to deal with any fears you have now so that you can concentrate on your labour when the time comes.

If you have specific worries, get as much information as you can about what lies ahead. If you are not sure how you will cope with the pain, for example, look into the different methods of pain relief that you can have. Don't rule anything out – even if you are keen to have a natural birth, it can be reassuring to know that you have access to medication if you need it.

## MENTAL PREPARATION

Take some time each day to contemplate the birth. Visualization can be very helpful: try to picture yourself in labour, adopting your preferred positions. Imagine yourself coping with the contractions – you may like to think of them as hurdles that you are leaping over or as powerful surges that are bringing you and your baby closer together. Think of your pelvic area opening and expanding, so that the baby passes more easily down the birth canal. Imagine your baby's arrival, and the joy that you will feel on seeing him or her. Think of the birth as an empowering rather than a worrying experience.

## PHYSICAL PREPARATION

In general, you want to feel as fit and healthy as possible. Get plenty of sleep and relaxation, so you start your labour feeling rested and mentally alert. If you are still working, consider starting your maternity leave (ideally you should leave work by week 34–36 so that you have time to prepare for the birth). Drink plenty of water to help your body expel any toxins. Eat healthily and regularly; you will find it easier to digest your food if you eat little and often. Eat plenty of complex carbohydrates, such as wholegrain bread and rice, in order to stock up your energy reserves. Make sure you eat iron-rich foods and protein each day, and include a wide range of different fruit and vegetables, to be sure that you are getting a full spectrum of nutrients.

Practising yoga or Pilates will help to enhance your suppleness and general health. It is also a good idea to practise your preferred positions for the labour, and to take a short walk each day to maintain your fitness.

## BREATHING EXERCISES

Controlling your breathing will help enormously at the birth. You will be taught breathing techniques at your antenatal classes, and you should practise these in advance. What you are aiming to avoid is the 'over-breathing' that results when we are tense and panicky – sucking air into our lungs and letting out short, sharp gasps. This will soon exhaust you, and fail to give yourself and your baby plenty of oxygen to cope with the birth.

Any breathing exercises you are given will focus on keeping your breathing steady and rhythmic. The in-breath should not be longer than the out breath; if anything, aim for the reverse. Try these simple exercises:
- Breathe in through your nose and out through your mouth, keeping your mouth soft. Try making a noise such as "Aaaaaaah" as you breathe out.
- As you breathe in, count slowly to three or four. Then do the same as you breathe out.

When it comes to pushing the baby out, you may automatically hold your breath as you push. This can hurt

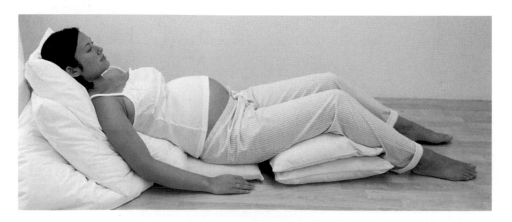

*Do not lie flat on your back at this stage of pregnancy. Prop yourself up on plenty of cushions and place another pillow or two under your knees. Alternatively, lie on your side with your uppermost leg resting on a cushion.*

your throat, and you should never hold your breath and push for as long as possible, which is sometimes advised, as this is tiring and oxygen-depleting. The better option is to take a deep breath as you feel a contraction starting, then breathe or blow out slowly as you push down.

If you feel the urge to push before the cervix is fully dilated, help to stop yourself from doing this as follows: give four short pants as a contraction arrives, then a quick in-breath, followed by four more pants. Breathe normally between contractions.

## NATURAL THERAPIES FOR THE LAST WEEKS

A traditional herbal preparation for labour is raspberry leaf tea (see page 60), while perineal massage helps to improve the stretchability of the skin (see pages 88–9). It can be very helpful to see an acupuncturist who specializes in pregnancy. Specific points can be used to strengthen the emotions and help you to prepare for the birth. Your acupuncturist may also be willing to teach you and your partner about acupressure points to press during labour.

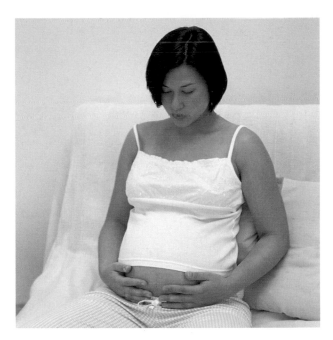

*Practise breathing techniques learned at antenatal classes every day, so that they become automatic.*

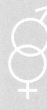

### NATURAL REMEDY BIRTH KIT

The following natural remedies may be helpful to you during labour. Check with a qualified practitioner to ensure that you take remedies that are suitable for your individual needs. You should also discuss with your midwife any remedies you wish to bring into the delivery room, and they should be incorporated into your birth plan.

#### Essential oils

A mixture of 10 drops clary sage, 10 drops lavender and 5 drops jasmine in 100ml (3½fl oz) base oil makes a good massage oil for the lower back during labour; it can help to promote strong contractions as well as encouraging you to stay calm. Useful oils to burn in a vaporizer may include frankincense (for pain and hyperventilation), lavender (for anxiety), rose (for fear and doubt), ginger (for weariness) and chamomile (for irritability).

#### Herbal teas

Teas that may be helpful during labour include raspberry leaf (to promote regular contractions), chamomile, lime flowers or lemon balm (to induce relaxation), cramp bark (to release tension) and ginseng (to boost energy). Check that there are tea-making facilities in the delivery suite; if not, take two flasks of hot water and a cup.

#### Flower remedies

Gentle flower remedies can be very comforting: place a few drops in a glass of water and sip at intervals. Try Rescue Remedy for fear and panic; olive for exhaustion; or cherry plum if you start to feel that you cannot carry on with the labour.

#### Homeopathic remedies

See a homeopath for advice about remedies that may be helpful to take before, during and after labour. He or she may recommend arnica (for bruising), caulophyllum (to encourage regular contractions), nux vomica (for backache) or hypericum (to promote healing).

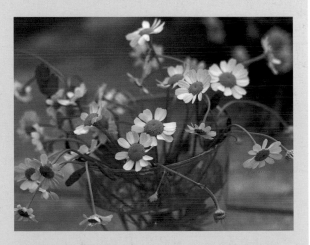

*Chamomile flowers are used to make calming tea or oil.*

# What your baby will need

Shopping is all part of the fun of expecting a baby. Unless you have already had a baby, you will need equipment for the nursery – a cot, a changing mat, a chest of drawers. You will also need a stock of clothes (remember that the baby will grow very quickly, so don't buy too many), nappies, toiletries and other items for the first few weeks. There are now plenty of natural and organic options available, so look out for these.

## WHAT TO BUY FOR...

### The nursery

- Cot with a drop-down side – make sure that you can drop down the side with one hand only (you may be holding your baby with your other arm).
- You may like to buy a Moses basket for the first four months or so. This is transportable so you will be able to move it around easily. It is a good idea to buy a stand to put the basket on at night. This means that you won't have to stoop to pick up the baby.
- Well-fitting new mattress for the cot and basket.
- Two cotton cellular blankets – these keep the baby warm, but not overheated.
- Linen, including cotton, fitted bottom sheets. Note that the baby will not need a pillow and must not have a duvet before the age of 12 months.
- Thick, dark curtains for daytime naps.
- Nursery thermometer – to monitor the temperature.
- A chair for you or your partner, or a small sofa.
- Changing table.
- A chest of drawers for clothes and nappies.
- Smoke alarm in or just outside the baby's room.
- Nightlight and baby monitor – check you have enough sockets.

### The kitchen or utility room

- Kitchen paper and disinfectant spray and wipes for cleaning surfaces.
- Check that washing machine, tumble dryer, washing line, clotheshorse and pulley are working properly. There will be a lot more washing than you are used to once the baby arrives. Make sure that you do not use biological washing powders since these may irritate a baby's sensitive skin.

### Feeding your baby

- Breast pads to catch leaks.
- Herbal nipple cream.
- Breast pump for expressing milk; for when you are somewhere where it would be difficult to breastfeed; this also allows your partner to feed the baby.
- Formula milk (organic varieties are available) and feeding bottles as standby.
- Bottle brush and teat brush.
- Sterilizing equipment (unless you just use boiling water). See pages 136–7.
- Bottle holders and carriers.
- Old towels to protect your clothes while feeding.

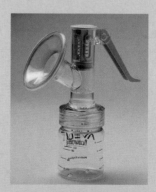
*A manual breast pump*

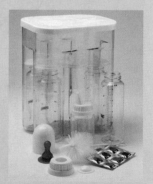
*Sterilizing tank and tablets*

### Your baby's clothes

- Vests, body suits and sleep suits.
- Dungarees.
- Dresses.
- Cardigans – easier to put on than sweaters.
- Socks or booties.
- Mittens, if winter.
- Warm hat or sun hat, depending on the season.
- Muslin squares.
- An all-in-one suit for outdoor wear.
- Small lightweight blanket.

**Playtime**
- Music.
- Rattles and soft toys.
- A ball.
- Mobile (to hang above cot).

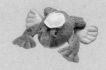

**Bathing your baby**
- Baby bath (choose from options that are used on or in an adult bath, and others that have their own stand).
- Natural baby soap, shampoo, lotion and oil, free from any harsh perfumes or colourings.
- Baby wipes for when you are out only (otherwise use water or lotion as the gentle, eco-friendly option).
- Cotton wool.
- Large tissues.
- Nappies and related accessories (see pages 138–9).
- Gentle herbal creams and oils for dealing with nappy rash (avoid using talc, see pages 138–9).
- Baby scissors or nail clippers.

**Your baby's health**
- Forehead strip thermometer.
- Basic first-aid kit and book.
- Gripe water.
- Herbal, homeopathic or conventional treatment for colic.
- Infant paracetamol syrup.
- Infant medicine spoon.
- Cough and cold treatments for infants.

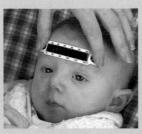

*A strip thermometer*

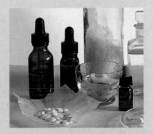

*Homeopathic remedies*

**Going out and about**
- Car seat – this must be correctly fitted; do not buy second-hand.
- Travel cot (or you can use a Moses basket).
- Lie-down baby buggy with transparent rain cover, or a pram (some are fitted with a removable carrycot to use as a bed, initially).
- Pram or buggy accessories, such as linen, cellular blankets, rain cover, parasol.
- Bag that is large enough to contain everything you need for feeding and changing your baby.
- A changing mat that you can put down anywhere on a table or on a floor.

- List of useful telephone numbers, such as your doctor's and health visitor's.

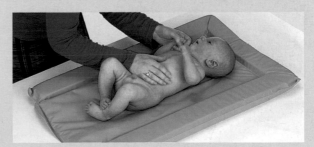

*Changing mat*

**Sources for everything you need**
Getting ready for a baby can be expensive, but there is no need to buy everything new. Shop around, and consider all the following sources:
- Friends and relatives.
- Charity shops and good second-hand shops.
- Magazines and direct-mail catalogues.
- The Internet.
- Large pharmacies and supermarkets (which often sell baby items more cheaply).

Remember that you are likely to be given outfits by friends and relatives. A close friend or relative who has recently had a baby may offer to pass on clothes and equipment that are no longer needed, especially if they are not planning another child.

**REMEMBER**
- Do not buy second-hand electrical equipment.
- If you are given or buy second-hand goods, make sure that they have been painted recently and do not contain leaded paint.
- Check catches, locks and hooks for safety.
- All clothes and linen should be washable and suitable for a tumble dryer.
- Cotton and light soft wools are kinder to the skin than synthetics.
- Avoid lots of buttons.
- Make sure that clothes are big enough to contain a nappy (diaper).

# Before the birth

As the birth approaches, your baby will be monitored as part of your continuing antenatal care. During the last month of your pregnancy, you will probably visit your antenatal clinic once a week for the usual blood and urine tests and weight check. In addition, your baby's heartbeat will be checked at each visit, and he or she will also be checked over to ensure that growth and movement are progressing normally.

You and your baby will be assessed for labour by the following criteria:

- Just how well the baby is likely to stand up to the testing rigours of labour and delivery – this is assessed by checking the baby's general well-being and heartbeat.
- Whether or not the baby is in the right position for a normal vaginal delivery.
- Whether or not the baby will be able to negotiate the birth canal – this is determined by assessing both the size of the baby's head and the size of the mother-to-be's pelvis.

A Caesarean section will be considered:

- If the baby's head is thought to be too large in relation to your pelvis.
- If he or she is in a position that will make it hard to navigate the birth canal.
- If there are likely to be any other complications during the delivery.

## THE POSITION FOR BIRTH

When discussing the baby's position for birth, medical staff will talk about the lie, the presentation and the position. These all mean different things.

### The baby's 'lie'

When doctors and midwives use the term 'lie', they are referring to the way that the baby is lying in the mother's body. This term describes the relationship between the spine of the baby and the spine of the mother – the north-south axis. The baby may be lying in a longitudinal (vertical) lie with the head up or head down, or across the mother's body in a transverse (horizontal) lie.

Nearly all babies before the 32nd week change the way they are facing frequently, so yours may be in the breech position when you have your antenatal check-ups: this is a longitudinal lie with the head uppermost and the buttocks down. After the 32nd week, most babies turn to the head-down position. About 3 per cent of babies,

however, remain in the breech position. Another 1 per cent of babies assume a transverse lie, in which the baby lies across the uterus. You can see all of these positions clearly in the illustrations.

Babies who are in a breech position or transverse lie may suffer some difficulties during a vaginal delivery, so special checks are made beforehand. In particular, it needs to be established whether or not the mother's pelvis is large enough to accommodate the baby comfortably. If the pelvis is not large enough, then a Caesarean delivery is advised. This is always the case with a transverse lie, but it may be that a breech baby is able to be delivered vaginally.

It is important to know if there is an underlying reason for the baby assuming the wrong lie. For example, the placenta may be in a position that makes it impossible for the baby to assume a head-down position, or there may be some other obstruction – such as a fibroid, for example – in the mother's uterus. In these cases, a Caesarean delivery will be carried out.

### The baby's presentation

This describes what part of the baby is at the pelvic brim before the delivery – that is, the part of the baby to be born first. Most babies adopt what is known as the vertex presentation. In this posture, the baby's head is well flexed, with the chin on the chest. This means that the vertex (crown) of the head is the part touching the cervix and will be born first.

A tiny number of babies – no more than 0.3 per cent – present their face or brow first. These presentations are known as face presentation or brow presentation. Face presentations are able to be delivered vaginally, but only if the back of the baby's head is facing the mother's spine. Brow presentations, however, are always delivered by Caesarean section because the baby cannot fit into the birth canal.

### The baby's position

A baby's position describes the way the baby is facing as birth approaches. If he or she is facing towards the mother's spine, the position is said to be anterior and labour is likely to be easier, although that is not always the case. If the baby is facing outwards, with the back of its head to the mother's spine, the position is said to be posterior. In this case, labour may be slower, and the mother is more likely to experience severe backache during labour.

## YOUR BABY'S POSITION

It can be hard to visualize the difference between a breech, transverse and face presentation. These illustrations show the various positions that a baby can adopt within the uterus in the last days before birth. All of them are perfectly comfortable for the baby, and none should cause undue discomfort to the mother.

### NORMAL POSITION

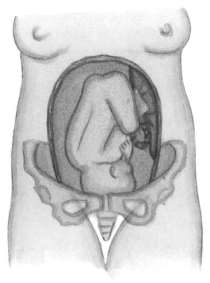

Here the baby is in the normal 'head-first' position, ready for the delivery. He or she is lying slightly to the right and is facing the mother's spine. The baby's chin is tucked into the chest, so that the narrowest part of the head will be born first.

### BREECH POSITION

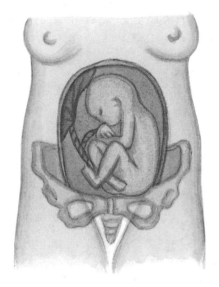

This baby is in the full, bottom-first breech position, with head up and legs crossed in front. Breech babies can have their legs extended up, so that their feet are in front of the face, or have one or both legs dropping down.

### TRANSVERSE LIE

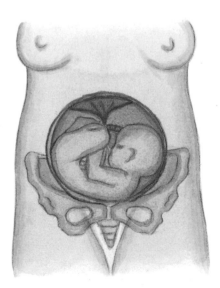

In a transverse lie, the baby is across the uterus. This means that his shoulder would come out first if a vaginal delivery were attempted. A baby can sometimes be encouraged to shift position, but, if this fails, a Caesarean section will be needed.

### FACE-DOWN PRESENTATION

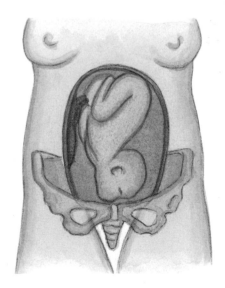

Here the baby is in the head-first position, but the neck is not tucked into the chest as in the normal position. Instead, the neck is extended so that the face is presented first. A midwife will assess whether or not a vaginal delivery is possible.

# Going into labour

There are three main stages of labour: the cervix dilating (opening up) to let the baby through; the actual birth itself; and the delivery of the placenta. Much more about these stages is explained over the following pages.

Women can find it hard to judge whether or not they have gone into labour. If you are in any doubt, you can contact your midwife at any time. You can also ring the hospital if you are not sure whether or not you should go in. There are three signs that indicate that labour is imminent or has started:

- A pinkish 'show' of mucus.
- The breaking of the waters.
- Contractions that last for 40 seconds or more, becoming more regular and pronounced.

## A 'SHOW'

The first sign that labour is imminent is usually the show. This occurs when the plug of mucus sealing the cervix is released. The show appears as a mucous vaginal discharge, which may be tinged with blood. It can happen several days before contractions start, or it may coincide with the breaking of the waters. It often goes unnoticed.

## THE BREAKING OF THE WATERS

The membranes surrounding the baby can rupture at the start of labour, shortly before it or at the end of the first stage. This is known as the breaking of the waters, and it is painless. Once this happens, you should go to hospital, or call your midwife if you are having a home birth.

Normally, waters break with an unmistakable gush of liquid. Sometimes there is a less obvious breaking that may be confused with the incontinence that is common in late pregnancy. Contact your midwife if you are unsure. In some cases, the waters break spontaneously but labour does not start. Most hospitals will admit you if this happens because the baby is no longer protected from infection and labour needs to be induced. Occasionally, however, the hole in the membrane seals itself over and the pregnancy continues. Sometimes the waters may be ruptured by the obstetrician using a probe. This may be done when the birth is being induced, as it can encourage contractions to start.

*Women may mistake the breaking of the waters for incontinence. Call your midwife if you think that you are in labour but cannot tell for certain.*

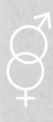

### THE WATERS
The term 'waters' refers to the liquid contained within the membranes. This amniotic fluid is a clear, yellowish liquid that contains the baby's urine and dead skin cells. Breaking the waters means breaking the membranes that surround and protect the baby in the uterus.

The baby depends for his or her well-being on the amniotic fluid. It has several functions:

- It enables the baby to turn and move his or her limbs easily.
- It serves to extend the uterus so that the walls do not exert any pressure upon the growing baby.
- It guarantees a constant temperature for the baby, which is the mother's body temperature.
- It absorbs the baby's waste products.
- It acts as a shock absorber, and so protects the baby from the impact if the mother falls or receives a jarring blow to the abdomen.

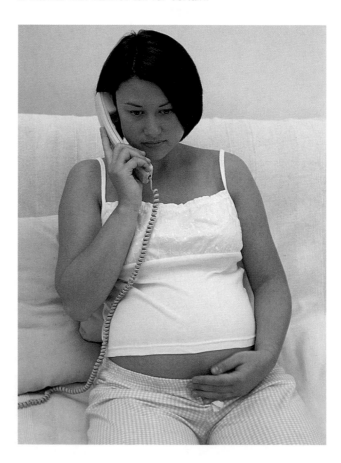

## CONTRACTIONS

Many women experience small, irregular contractions throughout pregnancy. Towards the end of pregnancy these become more pronounced, when they are known as Braxton Hicks contractions. They can be painful but are irregular and do not cause the cervix to dilate – so you are not in labour. With Braxton Hicks contractions, the uterus may contract every 20 minutes or so for about 20–30 seconds. By contrast, the birth contractions felt during the first stage of labour last for 40–60 seconds, and become more powerful. This is the time to telephone the hospital to tell them that you are on your way. It will help if you have noted down the frequency and length of the contractions.

## GOING TO HOSPITAL

Take your notes, birth plan and overnight bag with you. When you arrive at hospital, you will go through the normal admissions procedure and will then be taken to the labour ward, where your pulse, temperature and blood pressure will be checked and you will be examined externally and internally in order to judge the baby's position and see how far the cervix has dilated.

| HOW LONG DOES LABOUR LAST? | | |
| --- | --- | --- |
| | **First birth** | **Subsequent births** |
| 1st stage | 4–24 hours | 2–12 hours |
| 2nd stage | ½–2 hours | 10 minutes–1½ hours |
| 3rd stage | 10 minutes–1½ hours | 10 minutes–1½ hours |

When you go to the delivery room depends on how dilated you are, the baby's condition, and what space there is in the hospital. You may be allowed to make the delivery room a little more personal if you have arranged this beforehand – for example, plugging in a portable stereo or setting up an electric aromatherapy burner. These things should have been noted on your birth plan after discussion with the midwife, though there may not be time to carry this out if you are admitted as an emergency.

A team of midwives will provide all your medical care during labour, and will deliver your baby and check you are both well after delivery. Doctors are on duty for much of the day and night to assist if complications occur.

## THE SIGNS AND STAGES OF LABOUR

As already explained, there are three signs that herald the start of labour, and three stages to labour itself. The three warning signs may occur separately or in combination. So, you may be in the first stage of labour, with strong contractions lasting 40 seconds or more, even though the waters have not broken. The artworks below show how the cervix widens during labour. Shortly before labour begins, the cervix starts to shorten in response to the contractions. A partially dilated cervix, encouraged by the pressure of the baby's head, indicates that labour is well under way. By the time the cervix has dilated enough to allow the baby's head through into the vagina, the second stage of labour has been reached – this stage lasts from when the cervix is fully dilated until the birth of the baby. The third stage of labour is the delivery of the placenta.

### WHAT HAPPENS TO THE CERVIX BEFORE AND DURING LABOUR

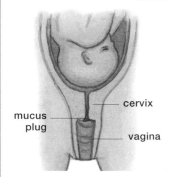

mucus plug — cervix — vagina

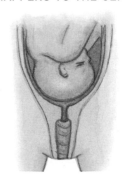

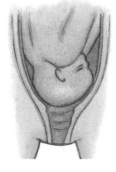

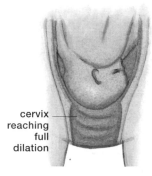

cervix reaching full dilation

*Here the neck of the uterus – the cervix – remains closed. It is sealed by a plug of mucus, which protects the baby from infection. When this is released, labour is near.*

*The mucus plug is released before labour – this is the 'show', one of the early signs that labour is near or has started. When the contractions begin, the cervix becomes shorter.*

*The cervix now starts to dilate (open). This is the first stage of labour, which can last many hours. A normal rate of dilation is judged to be about 1cm (⅖in) an hour, but this varies.*

*As the cervix reaches full dilation (10cm/4in), ready for the baby to pass down into the vagina, you are in a brief period called the transitional stage, just prior to the second stage of labour – the birth.*

# Pain relief and monitoring

The key to having as fulfilling a labour experience as possible is to keep an open mind and to be well informed beforehand about the signs of impending labour, how your labour is likely to be managed, the type of pain relief you would ideally like and all the options available.

**COMPLEMENTARY PAIN RELIEF**

There are many natural, drug-free methods that can help to ease the pain of labour and birth. Some of these work by stimulating the release of endorphins, the body's natural painkillers. To use some of these methods, you may need to have a complementary therapist with you in the delivery room. If you do, then this should be noted on your birth plan, along with details of any natural remedies you want to use.

Make sure that any therapist treating or helping you in the delivery room is fully experienced in dealing with labour and birth. Also, any therapies that you use must be ones that you are already familiar with and have had some success with before, so you know what to expect

**ORTHODOX PAIN RELIEF**

| Method | Stage of labour | How given | Does it work? | Side effects |
|---|---|---|---|---|
| **Gas and air** | 1st, 2nd | You breathe in from a mouthpiece | Up to a point – gives only limited relief from pain | May make you feel light-headed or drowsy. It is difficult to put your breathing techniques into practice while using mask |
| **Pethidine** | 1st | Injection either into a vein in the arm or into a muscle in the buttock | Timing is crucial – if given too early, effects may wear off; if too late, can prevent you pushing and can affect baby | May necessitate forceps delivery if it affects your ability to push. May make you feel drowsy and/or sick. The baby may be drowsy and slow to breathe |
| **Epidural** | 1st, and if Caesarean delivery | Injected into epidural space between spinal cord and backbone of lumbar region | Usually very effective but occasionally does not work | Chances of forceps delivery and episiotomy are higher if you have an epidural. Necessitates continuous fetal monitoring. You may feel numbness in legs for some time after delivery. May cause headache |
| **Pudendal nerve block** | 2nd, if forceps delivery is indicated | Injection through wall of vagina | Not always | None |
| **Transcutaneous Electrical Nerve Stimulation (TENS)** | 1st, 2nd | Electrodes attached to back, and a low-frequency current directed by mother | Not always | None – often recommended by complementary therapists |
| **General anaesthetic** | If Caesarean delivery | Injection | Yes | Recovery is often slow |

and are confident that they may have some effect. Below is a list of some common drug-free approaches:

- **Positions** Moving around and trying different positions – leaning against your partner or a wall, for example – will often bring relief (see also pages 120–3).
- **Water** Immersion in warm water is often relaxing, as the warmth is soothing and the water helps to take the body's weight. Find out well in advance about birthing pool options in your chosen place of delivery.
- **Massage** Effective for relieving discomfort and promoting calm, massage can easily be done by your birth partner. Massaging the lower back can be especially effective. To promote relaxation, stroke gently but firmly with the flat of the hand, working towards the heart. Using lavender oil will help to ease pain, while mandarin will lift the spirits.
- **Visualization/meditation** Practise well in advance. Simple approaches include imagining a scene such as a peaceful, sunny beach as contractions begin.
- **Acupuncture** This can be used to control various aspects of labour, from calming fears to easing backache. For the latter, needles can be inserted at points in the lower back. Needles can also be attached to an electrical device called an acutens machine, letting you control the stimulation level yourself.
- **TENS** (Trans-cutaneous Electrical Nerve Stimulation). This straddles orthodox and natural approaches (see table opposite). It uses a small electronic device attached to electrodes placed either side of the spine. Electric current is used to block pain impulses travelling along nerves and to stimulate endorphins.

## MONITORING THE BABY

With each contraction, the blood vessels supplying your baby with oxygen narrow, forcing the baby to hold its breath. Some babies cannot hold their breath for long and will become short of oxygen (distressed). If this happens for too long, they could suffer permanent damage or die.

During labour, the baby's heartbeat is monitored by the midwife, to detect any distress. In a low-risk pregnancy, a baby may be monitored for short spells by placing a Pinard stethoscope or an electronic ultrasound device on the mother's abdomen. In high-risk pregnancies, doctors may recommend continuous fetal monitoring during the latter part of the first stage of labour. There are two methods of continuous heart monitoring: external and internal.

In external monitoring, two belts are placed around the mother's abdomen. One holds the instrument that records the tightness and stretch of the abdomen during contractions, allowing the length and frequency of contractions to be measured. The other belt holds a transducer, which records the baby's heart rate. The belts are attached to a monitor, which records details of the baby's heartbeat and the mother's contractions.

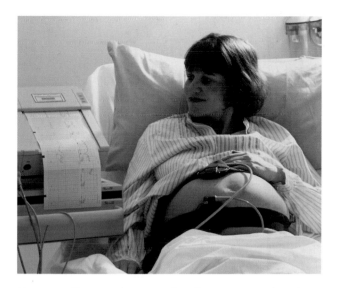

*Here, an ultrasound scanner has been strapped to the mother's abdomen to monitor her baby's heartbeat.*

With internal monitoring, once the cervix has dilated, a fetal scalp electrode is passed up through the woman's vagina and the end-point (a probe with a clip on the end) is fixed under the skin of the baby's scalp or buttocks. This allows a continuous read-out of the baby's heartbeat. If it slows for more than a minute or two, medical intervention may be needed.

If there is any sign of distress, a blood specimen can be obtained through a prick in the baby's scalp – fetal scalp sampling. The specimen's acidity reveals the degree of distress. If it is extreme, then immediate delivery, probably by Caesarean, will be carried out.

### DEALING WITH MONITORING

While monitoring is highly advantageous for the baby's health, the machinery needed can create a clinical atmosphere. It may also mean that the mother cannot move about freely during labour and often requires her to lie down at an angle that is somewhat unnatural and difficult for childbirth. Always tell medical staff how you feel about the monitoring process so that the most satisfactory compromise can be reached.

However, there are active birth positions that you may be able to get into when attached to a monitor. Adjust the bed head to a comfortable sitting position, usually around a 25° angle. Bend your legs alternately for about 10 minutes, placing the sole of the foot of the bent leg against the inner thigh of the straight leg. You could also kneel on the bed and lean against the angled bed head, using pillows for support. Another position is resting on your side with one bent leg above the other and a pillow between your knees. If possible, swap between these positions every half hour or so, to create a rhythm that helps to relieve contraction pain.

# The first stage of labour

During the first stage of labour, you should feel free to follow your instincts and do whatever feels right for you. You may find yourself rocking or swaying during contractions. Many women like to take a bath, finding the sensation of water to be pleasantly soothing.

Move around and try out new positions until you find the one or two that seem most comfortable. Any of the positions shown here may be right for you.

A lot of women like to keep moving around during the first stage of labour, getting into their favourite position each time a new contraction starts. Take one contraction at a time, and breathe your way through it, perhaps using imagery to help you. For example, you could try to visualize your cervix opening out like a flower.

### THE TRANSITIONAL STAGE

This is the term for the short period of time at the end of the first stage of labour, just before moving into the second stage. It is the shortest part of labour, but it can be very intense and contractions can feel even more painful and seem to be absolutely relentless.

You may feel discouraged and find yourself not wanting to go on for much longer without additional pain relief. You may also be very emotional and perhaps irritable or bad-tempered. Your legs may start shaking and you might shiver; you may even need to vomit.

You may also get an urge to push, or bear down, though you shouldn't do this until the midwife has examined you and has confirmed that your cervix is fully dilated. Panting a little may help you resist the urge.

Whenever you feel that you just can't go on, remember that your baby will be born soon. Keep telling yourself to hang on, stay calm, and all will be well.

### GOOD POSITIONS IN TRANSITION

It is difficult to find a comfortable position when you are in transition. Any position that you have found helpful up to this point is suitable for use now. You may like to kneel forward over a pile of cushions, or you may prefer to stand, sit, squat, or be held in a supported squat.

If the cervix has not yet fully dilated and you feel the urge to bear down, try kneeling on all fours: put your head down against the floor and your bottom up in the air. This position uses the force of gravity to help slow the baby down, while the cervix continues to dilate. This position also takes pressure off your lower back.

---

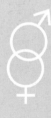

**HELPING SOMEONE GIVE BIRTH**
Remember that labour can be a traumatic and difficult time for a woman, so be prepared to deal with any strange or aggressive behaviour without getting offended. If she tells you to go away, stand aside, but do not go too far away. However useless you feel, you do have an important role.

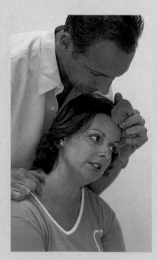

*Simple actions such as sponging your partner's face and holding her hand can help a lot. Don't be surprised if she shouts at you – and at anyone else around.*

- Try to help her to relax, especially between the contractions.
- Help her to cool down with a water spray or moist sponge if she's hot.
- Wipe away perspiration from her face.
- Encourage her by telling her she's doing fine, never criticize her.
- Be alert to her moods and adapt to them.
- If she feels sick and says that she wants to throw up, get her a bowl quickly.
- If her legs begin to tremble, hold her legs firmly and offer her a pair of socks in order to keep them warm and so help her circulation.
- If she has backache, massage her lower back and offer her a hot-water bottle.
- If she says she wants to push or she starts to grunt and make pushing motions, tell the midwife immediately.
- Once the midwife has told her that she is fully dilated and she can push, let the midwife guide her through the pushing stage. Always do what the midwife tells you.
- Drink lots of water to keep yourself hydrated.

## SIT

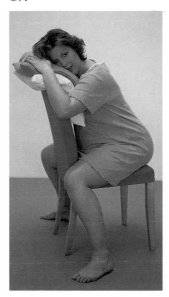

*Sit astride a chair, facing its back, with knees apart and your back straight. Put a cushion against the back of the chair and lean against it. In this position, your body is vertical yet completely supported, and your pelvis is kept open.*

## STAND

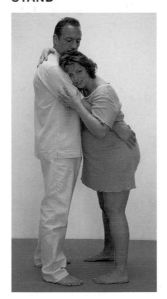

*Stay upright and lean slightly forwards against your birth assistant. The downward force of gravity stimulates contractions and encourages the baby's descent. You may find it helpful to circle your hips. Your birth assistant can massage your lower back in this position, or rock you gently.*

## KNEEL

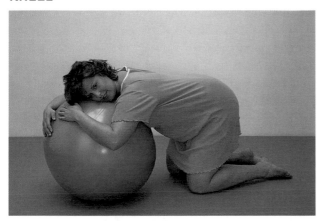

*Kneel down and support yourself by leaning forwards against a nearby piece of sturdy furniture, over a pile of cushions or a big bean bag. You can also use a birthing ball for this.*

## SQUAT

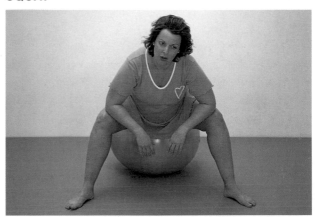

*Squat on a low stool or birthing ball. This position tends to intensify contractions, as well as allowing the pelvis to open widely. It also encourages the baby's descent.*

## KNEEL ON ALL FOURS

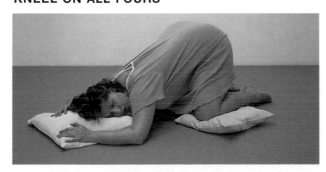

*Kneel on all fours and rock back and forth during contractions. If they are very intense, kneel with your head against the floor and bottom in the air. Try moving your hips around, too.*

## LIE DOWN

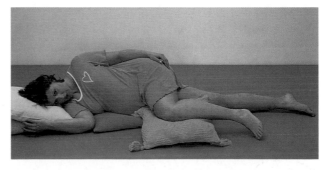

*You may feel like lying down, particularly if you are getting tired. Try lying on your side, with your 'bump' well supported on cushions. It is not a good idea to lie on your back for any length of time, although this is fine for when you are being examined.*

# The second and third stages

When the cervix is fully dilated (about 10cm/4in), you have entered the second stage of labour. The second stage can be over in minutes or it may take up to two hours. It ends with the birth of the baby. Second-stage contractions are typically very strong, with the whole body engaged in a massive involuntary urge to bear down. This is a reflex, caused by the baby's head pressing on the pelvic floor and the rectum. Even if you had read nothing about the birth, you would know instinctively when to take a deep breath, thus lowering your diaphragm and exerting pressure on the uterus, which helps to push the baby out. Some women find the second stage easier than the first, although it may be difficult, especially if the baby is large or there are worries about tearing.

## BEST POSITIONS FOR BIRTH

Pushing is harder work if you are lying on your back, because you are pushing the baby uphill. An upright, or semi-upright, position is therefore best for delivery, as gravity will help your efforts. Your pelvis should be open, and your pelvic floor and vaginal opening needs to be relaxed. Many women move about and change position throughout the second stage of labour, eventually finding the best position for them for birth. The following positions, shown opposite, are all suitable for the delivery:

- **Lying down** This position is good if you are feeling exhausted. Lie on your side with your head resting on a couple of pillows. Keep your legs open by holding the knee – your birth assistant can do this for you.

- **Sitting** Here, the woman sits propped up with plenty of bulky cushions, with her knees bent and apart, and her head dropped forwards towards her chest. This position lets her see the baby being born. However, it is an unnatural position for birth and unhelpful for the baby, so it is not the best one to use.

- **Kneeling** Many women choose to give birth in this position. Kneel on all fours, leaning over a bean bag or large cushion. The midwife receives the baby from behind. A kneeling position eases pressure on the perineum, allowing the soft tissues to expand and stretch as the baby is born.

- **Squatting** This is often found to be a good position. You can squat either while being supported from behind by one helper, or while being supported on either side by two helpers. Squatting opens up the pelvis to its maximum, relaxes the pelvic floor and uses the force of gravity. If squatting with one helper, your helper should stand, or preferably sit, behind you in a firm and stable stance. He should support you by taking your weight on his arms. Surrender completely to the contraction, bending your knees and spreading your feet apart so that the pelvis opens. This position usually encourages a rapid birth and is particularly suitable if there is any reason to speed up delivery, as in cases of fetal distress or a long labour. It is also helpful in a breech birth.

## YOUR BABY EMERGES

Pushing a baby out is hard work. Try to do so smoothly and gradually, so all the vaginal muscles and tissues have the chance to stretch in order to allow the baby's head through without tearing or necessitating an episiotomy.

The first sign that the baby is entering the world is a bulging of the perineum and the anus. More and more of the baby's head then appears at the vaginal opening, which is known as crowning, at which point you may feel a stinging sensation as the baby pushes against your vagina. This sensation can be eased by deep breathing, or if an attendant holds a warm compress against the perineum, helping the tissues to stretch. Sometimes the baby will be born very quickly at this stage, with its head and body coming out in one contraction. The birth may also take place more slowly, over a number of contractions. Typically, as the baby's head emerges, it will turn its head to one side. Your contractions may cease briefly here, giving those attending you the chance to check that the umbilical cord is not wrapped around the baby's neck and, if it is, to reposition the cord more safely.

Your next contraction should see the baby's shoulders emerging, and once these are out, the rest of the baby's body will follow on swiftly, usually followed by gushing amniotic fluid.

### SPEED OF DELIVERY

How fast delivery occurs depends on your position and that of the baby's head, as well as its size. If it is slow and you are in a lot of pain, medical staff will help you breathe the baby out gently in order to avoid a tear. If it is felt that you are likely to tear badly, the doctor will perform an episiotomy.

## LYING

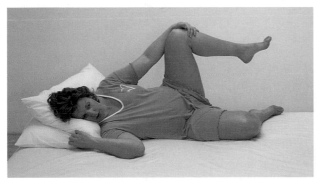

## SITTING

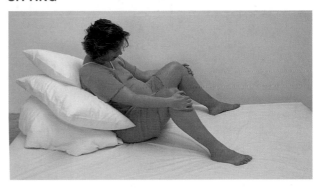

## KNEELING

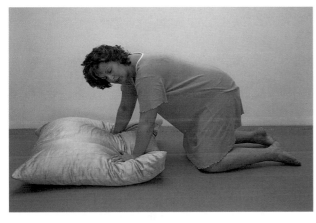

## A SUPPORTED SQUAT

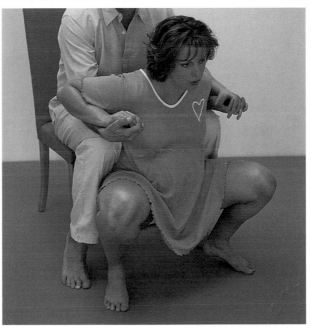

*These pictures show four principal positions commonly adopted during the second stage of labour and delivery. The woman should be made as comfortable as possible with supportive cushions and allowed to swap between positions – she needs to find what is best and most comfortable for her.*

### YOUR BABY HAS ARRIVED

Caregivers will typically wrap the baby up and let you hold her immediately. Your baby may be breathing and crying as soon as he or she emerges, and may start to suckle virtually straight away.

If you are delivering twins, the procedures are the same. However, a twin delivery is more risky and complex, for the babies and the mother. There is an increased risk of fetal distress, and the likelihood of a Caesarean is higher with a twin delivery than with a single baby.

### THE THIRD STAGE OF LABOUR

This stage occurs after delivery of the baby and is simply the expulsion of the placenta. When the baby is born, the uterus rests, but about 15 minutes later it starts to contract again, relatively painlessly, to expel the placenta and its membranes. You can help to push out the

*Be prepared for a turbulent mix of emotions once the birth is over – relief, joy, shock, exhaustion and tearfulness are all perfectly normal reactions.*

placenta yourself, both by squatting and also by putting the baby to the breast, which helps the uterus to contract. Medical staff will now carefully examine the placenta to make sure that absolutely all of it has been expelled, as leaving bits behind may lead to internal bleeding. Checks are then made for any large tears around the vulva area, which will have to be stitched.

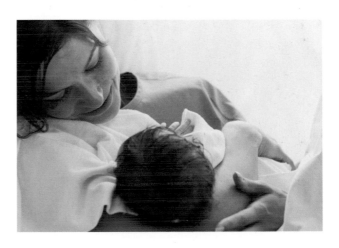

# Medical interventions

Sometimes births go slowly or other problems develop. Medical staff may intervene to hasten the birth if they think there is any danger to the mother or baby.

## DELIVERY BY FORCEPS

Forceps can be used to facilitate a speedier delivery. They look rather like big salad servers and are sometimes used to help the baby out in the second stage of labour, when the cervix is fully dilated and the baby's head has come down into the mother's pelvis but is not descending any further. They may also be used in cases of fetal or maternal distress. The forceps are easy to apply and cause no harm to the baby if applied properly, although the baby's head may be marked.

Your legs will be put in stirrups and a local anaesthetic injected into the perineum. An episiotomy (cut) is then done, and forceps inserted into the vagina and the blades cupped round the sides of the baby's head. The idea is that the mother then pushes, while the doctor pulls. Once the head is delivered, the forceps are removed and you can push the baby out normally.

## VENTOUSE EXTRACTION

More than one in ten deliveries now involve the use of ventouse ('vacuum extraction' in the US). Like forceps, it is used to help speed the delivery. A suction cap is attached to the baby's head and suction is used to pull the baby out gently with each contraction as you push.

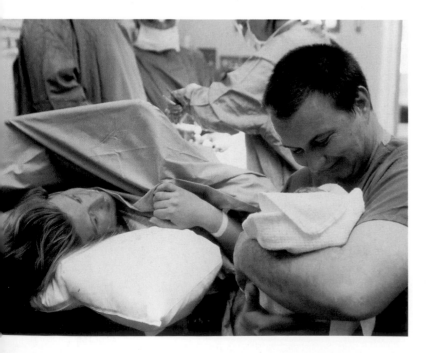

There are no risks to the baby and no drugs need to be used. The advantages of this method over forceps delivery is that the cervix does not need to be fully dilated, and it is perceived as a lesser intervention. The mother still has to do a fair measure of the pushing so she does not feel quite so outmanoeuvred by technology.

The disadvantage is that it can take time to apply enough suction. The baby may have a small bump on its head rather like a large bruised blister, which subsides after a day or two.

## INDUCTION OF LABOUR

Sometimes, labour may need to be artificially induced. This is done by breaking of the waters and by giving the mother drugs, vaginally or intravenously. An induction may be done for the following reasons:

- The baby is overdue and the placenta is becoming less able to supply his or her needs.
- Raised blood pressure in the mother.
- Pre-eclampsia.
- Rhesus incompatibility.
- Bleeding in late pregnancy.
- Diabetes.
- The baby has stopped growing.

## EPISIOTOMY

An episiotomy is a cut in the perineum. A local anaesthetic is given first, and then a cut is made – using scissors – into the skin and muscle at the lower end of the woman's vagina. After the birth, the cut is stitched up. Some people believe that a natural tear heals faster than a cut. An episiotomy may be needed in an assisted delivery, or if the woman is likely to be severely torn.

Getting into a good delivery position will help minimize the chances of episiotomy. If you would like to avoid having one, you should discuss this well in advance with the medical staff who are taking care of you and include it in your birth plan.

## CAESAREAN SECTION

A Caesarean is a major surgical procedure whereby both baby and placenta are delivered through a cut in the mother's abdomen rather than through the vagina. It may be done under general anaesthetic or after an epidural, in

*A delighted father holds his baby after birth by caesarian section. It takes a mother a little time to recover from this operation – as with any major surgery.*

which case the mother will be awake when her baby is delivered. It is possible to have your labour companion with you during this operation if you have an epidural, but not if you have a general anaesthetic.

There are two types of Caesarean section: elective (by choice) and emergency.

- **Elective Caesareans** These are planned during pregnancy, usually because there is a medical or obstetric complication which means that a vaginal delivery is considered unsafe. Occasionally, women choose to have their baby delivered by Caesarean because of a personal preference.
- **Emergency Caesareans** A Caesarean may need to be done following complications that occur during labour, when your baby has become distressed and needs to be delivered speedily and safely.

### Reasons for a Caesarean

There are many reasons why a Caesarean may be done. They include the following:

- If the baby is large and the mother's pelvis is small, making normal delivery virtually impossible.
- If the baby is premature, small or particularly vulnerable to distress.
- Pregnancies in which there is more than one baby.
- Babies who are in a position – such as a transverse lie – that makes normal delivery impossible.
- Inefficient contractions – which mean that the labour does not progress.
- Placental abruption, in which the placenta detaches itself from the wall of the uterus. This usually causes pain and bleeding, and necessitates the immediate delivery of the baby.
- Placenta praevia, in which the placenta is lying across the cervix and would be ruptured if labour were allowed to continue, causing dangerous bleeding, (known as antepartum haemorrhage).
- When the mother has a condition such as high blood pressure, pre-eclampsia or diabetes.
- When the umbilical cord has prolapsed and is presenting before the baby, obstructing the delivery.
- When an induction has not worked.
- If there are tumours such as fibroids or ovarian cysts, which will obstruct the baby's delivery.
- If the mother has had a pregnancy that ended in stillbirth, or if she has experienced a previous complicated and difficult delivery.
- If the baby becomes severely distressed.

### WHEN DOCTORS INTERVENE

Medical intervention in labour is becoming more common: about one in five births in the UK is by Caesarean delivery and the situation is similar in the USA. Some experts are concerned that medical staff can be too quick to intervene, and that some problems may resolve themselves naturally if allowed to do so. However, there is no doubt that intervention has saved the lives of many babies.

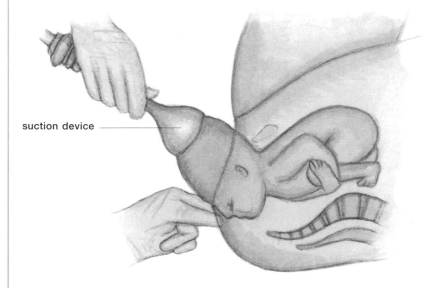

suction device

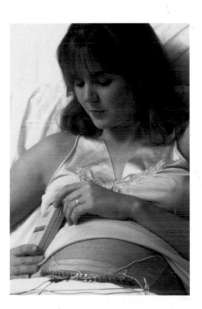

*Assisted delivery may be necessary if the labour is progressing very slowly, if the baby becomes distressed or if the mother becomes so exhausted that she can no longer push. Here, a ventouse attached to the baby's head is used to help bring it out of the birth canal.*

*This woman is using a TENS pain-relief machine to cope with post-Caesarean discomfort. The stitched scar is from the operation.*

# Checklist of common problems

The last few weeks of pregnancy can be quite uncomfortable, and you may long to get the birth over with. Just remember that each day is bringing you a day closer to holding your baby. You may still be suffering from minor ailments, such as haemorrhoids or backache, at this stage. Natural therapies can often alleviate the worst of your symptoms and can also help you to cope with any tension. They may also help your baby to be better prepared for the birth – by virtue of you yourself being more relaxed.

Always discuss any natural remedies that you wish to take with your midwife – you will see her every week during the last month of pregnancy, so you will have plenty of opportunity to discuss any plans, anxieties or problems. If you decide to consult a complementary practitioner, make sure that you see only qualified therapists who are experienced in treating pregnant women. If you have any symptoms that are severe, prolonged or concern you, contact your midwife or doctor straight away. See page 75 for a list of emergency warning symptoms.

**Breech baby**   Most babies are in the buttocks-down (breech) position before 32 weeks but most will turn so that they are head-down for the birth. If your baby is in the breech position after 32 weeks, he or she may well turn spontaneously before the birth. There are also several natural methods that may help to encourage a breech or transverse baby to turn. Do not try any natural therapies if you are having twins or if you are ill.

- Take an hour-long walk each day. This may encourage your baby to move to the head-down position. Practising some yoga positions – such as 'the cat' – may also encourage the baby to move.
- Spend some time each day visualizing your baby moving into the right position. Make sure that you are feeling relaxed and comfortable when you do this – slow your breathing down and let go of any tension in your body first.
- The homeopathic remedy pulsatilla is sometimes used to encourage a baby to turn. Do not be tempted to self-prescribe; see a qualified homeopath to ensure that the remedy is suitable for you and that you take the correct dosage, and so that the homeopath can monitor the outcome.
- Moxibustion is a traditional Chinese method for turning breech babies. It is supported today by a variety of complementary practitioners, although it should be noted that doctors now do not attempt to

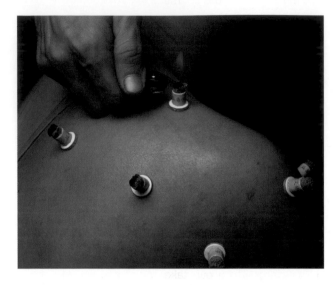

*In moxibustion, a tiny amount of burning moxa is placed on different energy points on the body. In pregnancy, the points most typically used are located on the toes.*

turn babies, as complications can result. Moxibustion involves lighting a stick of the herb moxa and holding it near acupuncture points on the outer corner of each little toe, or burning small amounts of the herb on the skin. The heat is said to stimulate the bladder energy channel, which is connected to the uterus. Moxibustion also has a general soothing effect. If you wish to try out moxibustion treatment, then you must seek the assistance of an experienced acupuncturist who is used to treating pregnant women, and do not attempt to do the treatment to yourself, or at home.

**Late baby**   Babies that are more than two weeks overdue are usually induced in hospital; induction may also be advised if your waters break early or you have high blood pressure. There are a number of natural methods that you can try if you have advance warning of an induction, but always talk to your midwife beforehand.

- Keep upright and keep moving around – activity can sometimes bring on contractions, but you should not overdo it.

> ❝ Natural therapies can often alleviate the worst of your symptoms and can also help you to cope with any tension you are feeling. ❞

- Make love. Having an orgasm can sometimes help to stimulate uterine contractions.
- Consult an acupuncturist: various points on the back can be stimulated, sometimes with electricity, in order to bring on contractions. You may need several treatments over the course of a week.
- See a reflexologist, who will work on various points on your feet.
- The homeopathic remedy caulophyllum is sometimes used to encourage contractions. However, you will need to see a qualified homeopath to ensure that this remedy is right for you, and so that your progress can be monitored.
- Try practising breathing techniques for relaxation, then visualize yourself going into labour. It can be helpful to do this daily.

**Fear and anxiety** Anxiety is a very common emotion for mothers-to-be. It is important that you discuss any specific worries that you have with your midwife. She may be able to put your mind at rest or advise you on any practical steps you can take. You might like to try the following suggestions:
- Practise relaxation techniques, such as yoga, Pilates, meditation or visualization. You may find it helps calm fears if you regularly visualize yourself and your baby surrounded by healing golden light.
- Consider complementary therapies, such as reiki, acupuncture or reflexology, all of which may help with stress or worry.

- Try Bach Flower Remedies, which are very gentle. Mimulus is good if you have specific, named fears, such as anxiety about the labour, while aspen is used for vague, unspecific fears. Red chestnut can be taken for excessive concern about the baby's well-being, and Rescue Remedy is excellent if you have moments of panic and tearfulness.
- Use essential oils such as lavender or rosewood, which can be very soothing in late pregnancy: use them in a burner or diluted in the bath or in a relaxing massage oil.

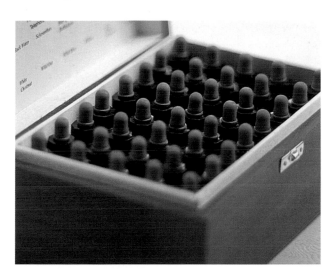

*Bach Flower Remedies can be an effective natural way to relieve anxiety and fear. Keep them in a special box, separated out so each one retains its healing properties.*

## Instant calm

If you are feeling anxious or fearful, try this simple exercise to release tension and calm yourself down.

It serves to activate the energy channel of the heart, and it can feel very soothing and loving.

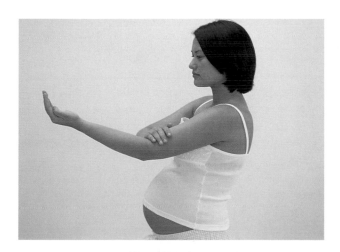

**1** Hold your left arm straight out in front of you. Keep it loose rather than taut, and drop your shoulders to release tension here. Gently cup your right hand around the upper arm, just above the elbow.

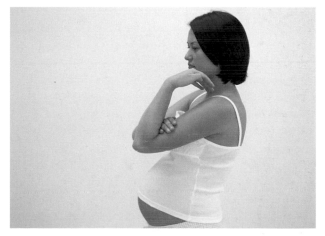

**2** Now, bring your forearm slowly towards your shoulder, until it rests upon your other hand. Breathe quietly for a few moments, focusing on your heart area, and feel a sense of release here.

# Common Qs and As

Q: I felt my contractions starting and my partner took me to the hospital but they sent me home again, saying I wasn't ready yet. How could that happen?

A: It is possible to have contractions that mimic those of labour but are shorter and less pronounced. Once the hospital checks you out, they can tell immediately by how dilated your cervix is whether or not you have started true labour.

Q: I was planning a natural, drug-free birth but now my baby is going to be induced as I am two weeks overdue. I have heard that the contractions are more intense after an induction. Is that true?

A: Not necessarily. It depends on the individual woman, the reasons for the induction, how overdue she is, the drugs used, and how your particular hospital manages labour in respect of pain relief. It is better to induce a birth than to let the baby stay too long in the uterus, because there comes a point when the placenta can no longer nourish the baby.

Q: I had a very drawn-out, painful birth with my first child. My consultant has offered me an elective Caesarean. Do you think that this is a good idea?

A: It depends on the reasons why this has been offered. If the consultant knows that you are facing another lengthy and painful delivery, clearly it is sensible to elect for a Caesarean. If, for example, your pelvis and birth canal are too narrow to deliver a baby vaginally, the baby must be born by Caesarean. If, on the other hand, you are being offered a Caesarean to put your mind at rest, it may be better to try for a natural delivery first and only then to go for a Caesarean if there appears to be no other alternative. So, ask your consultant exactly why you have been offered a Caesarean, think it over, and base your decision on his or her advice.

Q: I am keen to give birth naturally and without pain relief. To me, it will not be a real birth if the doctors take control. How can I make sure that that this does not happen?

A: If everything goes well, you will not need medical intervention. You can give yourself the best possible chance of a natural birth by preparing well, practising your breathing exercises regularly, and by stating your wishes on a birth plan.

However, you cannot guarantee that your delivery will be straightforward. If anything does go wrong, you would be well advised to take advantage of all the skills and technology that modern medicine can offer. In the end, it is more important that your baby comes into the world safe and healthy than that you have the childbirth experience you hoped for.

Q: My underlying fears about coping with the financial aspects of having a baby are really crowding in on me now that the birth is imminent. How on earth are we going to pay for everything that the baby will need?

A: First of all, it is natural to start obsessing over certain worries once the baby is due, as this is a vulnerable time for you. Just focus on the fact that the most important thing for your baby is that he or she is with you. Your baby does not need much: just to be warm, fed and looked after. Think of positive solutions to any worries, such as asking your midwife if there are any outlets in your area where you can buy decent second-hand items.

**Q**: My partner seems quite relaxed about giving birth, but she has said she wants me to be there. I am not sure if I can handle this.

**A**: Many men feel this way. Some men really cannot cope and it would be unwise to try to persuade them. A few men have said that they never felt the same way about their partners once they had seen them giving birth. For other men, however, seeing their partner give birth is an absolute highlight of their life.

Explain exactly how you feel to your partner. It may be that when the time comes, you do feel able to be there. Alternatively, you could promise to be nearby during her labour, even if you feel unable to be in the room. You should also suggest that she takes someone else to support her through the labour. This will take the pressure off you, and you may then feel able to be there for some of the time.

**Q**: I have just broken up with my partner even though I am 36 weeks pregnant. I know that our decision to split is right for both of us but I am dreading giving birth alone.

**A**: You do not have to be alone. You can elect for one of your friends, a sister or another member of your family to be there with you. You could investigate the possibility and cost of a private room after giving birth for you and your new baby.

Try to arrange for extra help at home after the birth. Is there anybody who could come to help you for a couple of weeks after the birth? If not, it is a good idea to have at least one visit a day from friends or relatives. You should also tell your midwife your situation, as she may be able to arrange extra help.

**Q**: I have been asked to take part in a research project during my pregnancy and labour. Do I have to agree to this?

**A**: Many maternity units are committed to ongoing research projects to improve standards of clinical care. You may be asked to take part, but you do not have to. Many units are responsible for training doctors and midwives who need to conduct normal deliveries under close supervision by experienced midwives. You may refuse this option, but many women welcome the support that students can give them during labour.

**Q**: I am a single mother who is expecting my second child. I am worried that there will be prejudice about this from some of the other women on the delivery ward and from the nurses. How can I best cope with this?

**A**: Many women now have children when they are single: you are unlikely to be an unusual case. Nobody will be surprised if your birth partner is a friend or relative rather than the father.

You may find it helpful to discuss your anxieties with your midwife, and to note on your birth plan that you would like as much privacy as possible. Take a friend or relative to support you through the labour. Above all, remember it is your life and your baby: be happy and proud of the decisions you have made.

# CHAPTER FIVE
# You and your new baby

" Your baby's needs are now the most important consideration in your life. "

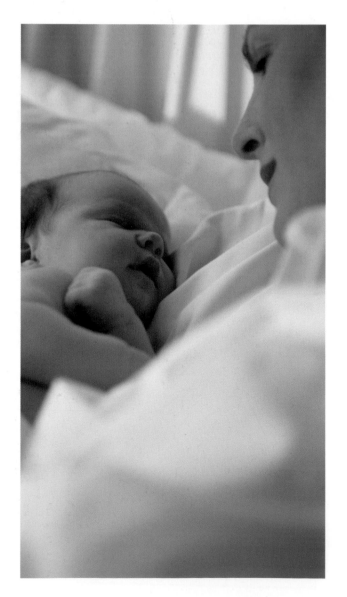

Your baby's feelings and needs are now the most important consideration in your life. When you offer your baby his or her very first feed, you are likely to experience a variety of emotions: joy, wonder, exhaustion and relief that all is well.

When you speak, your baby will recognize the distinctive rhythms of your voice, which he or she has heard for many months while growing inside you. He or she will be gazing at you, experiencing your smell, your look and the texture of your skin.

In turn, you and your partner are likely to spend many hours gazing at your baby, looking into his or her eyes, marvelling at the tiny fingers and toes, and the minute nails. You will be examining every curve of your baby's tiny body, every indentation, even the hairs on his or her head.

When you bath your baby for the first time, you may find that you naturally respond to his or her vulnerability with the gentlest touch. You will come to cherish the softness of your baby's skin and his or

*Newborn babies cannot see very far. At first, they can see what is immediately in front of them, but very little more than that.*

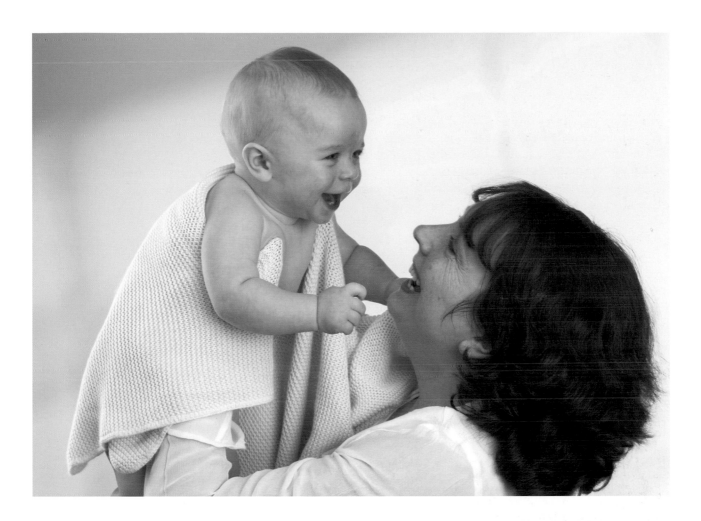

her natural helplessness, and you will want to do everything in your power to love and care for his or her various needs.

However much you love your baby though, you are likely to find that you experience some difficult emotions during these first weeks. Most women feel sad, anxious or overwhelmed at times – and everyone feels exhausted.

It is very important that you look after yourself as well as your baby. In particular, get as much sleep and rest as you can, whenever you can. Eat healthily and often, and try to get some fresh air every day. This will help you to cope with the inevitable challenges of looking after a small baby.

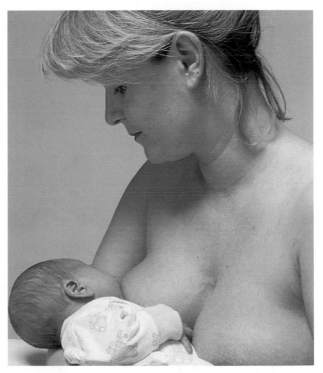

*Top: Enjoying – and making time for – having plenty of interaction and fun together is enormously important for both parent and baby.*

*Your baby will enjoy the physical comfort of being breastfed, and breastfeeding helps you to know that you are doing everything possible to meet his or her needs.*

# Meeting your new baby

At long last you are being handed your baby. This is the moment that you and your partner have been waiting for. Whatever difficulties you have faced during the pregnancy, whatever kind of labour and delivery you have had, all that is now behind you. This is the moment to savour for the rest of your life – the very beginning of your child's life and the start of your lives as parents.

If you have delivered your baby in hospital, you will probably be left alone with your partner and the baby for a while. This will depend partly on how well you and the baby have stood up to the rigours of the birth. At some point, your pulse and blood pressure will be checked and your temperature will be taken. You will be able to take a bath. The baby will be weighed and measured in length and head circumference, footprinted and given a name band. She will also be assessed according to the Apgar score (see box below).

The umbilical cord will be clamped and cut when it has stopped pulsating after the birth and the clamped stump at the baby's navel will be left to drop off of its own accord within the next few days. A small blood sample

*This is the moment that makes it all worthwhile – holding your lovely new baby. Medical staff will be sensitive and leave you alone with your baby as soon as possible.*

> **" This is the moment that makes it all worthwhile – holding your lovely new baby. "**

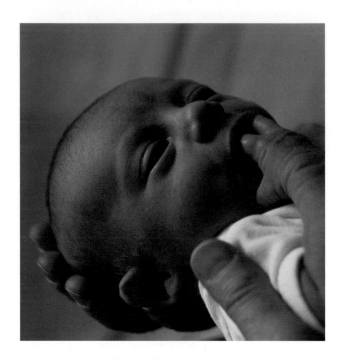

## THE APGAR SCORE

Soon after the birth, your baby will need to be cleaned, weighed and measured. A name band will be placed around his or her wrist if you are in hospital. The baby's health will be assessed a minute after the delivery. This is done using the Apgar score in which five factors are checked. Points are awarded from 0 to 2 for each of the five factors. The baby who scores 10 is in good general health; if your baby scores less than ten, he or she may need special care for a while. The test may be repeated after five minutes.

| SIGN | 0 POINT | 1 POINT | 2 POINTS |
|---|---|---|---|
| **Respiratory effort (breathing)** | None | Weak cry, slow breathing | Good strong cry |
| **Pulse (heart rate)** | None | Slow, under 100 beats per minute | Fast, over 100 beats per minute |
| **Colour (pallor)** | Blue or pale | Pink body with blue fingers and toes | All pink |
| **Muscular tone** | Limp | Some flexing of fingers and toes | Active: fingers and toes flexing well |
| **Response to stimuli (reflexes)** | No response | Grimace | Cry |

*One secure way of holding your newborn baby is to cradle him in your arms, in the crook of your elbow, making sure that his head is well supported.*

will be taken from the baby so that the Guthrie test can be done. This is used to detect phenylketonuria, a disease which causes mental impairment if left untreated. If the test is positive, the baby can be treated for the condition with complete success.

## MARKS AND RASHES

When your baby first arrives, you may notice a few minor bumps and wrinkles caused by the journey down the birth canal. He or she may even have a little bruise and the odd spot, rash or area where the skin tone is blotchy, while some newborns have puffy eyes. The baby may have enlarged breasts and genitals caused by hormonal fluctuations, which will settle soon after birth. This is all very normal.

There are certain other skin marks that are more permanent. These include pale pink 'stork bite' markings on the face or neck that disappear within the first year; blue spots common on darker-skinned babies that fade away; and 'strawberry' birthmarks that start as red dots and may get larger within the first year, normally disappearing by the age of about five. Larger flat areas of red or purple known as 'port wine stains' are permanent – seek a doctor's advice about these.

## INITIAL BONDING

Some new parents immediately experience a huge well of love for their newborn. Many women will have started the bonding process with their baby many weeks before giving birth, perhaps even from the first scan or earlier. For others, and for many fathers, too, the bonding process may take longer.

As you look at your baby in the first minute of new life, you will probably feel overwhelmed with emotion. You may find yourself simultaneously full of pleasure and weariness, curiosity and relief. Your baby will be looking at you, and taking in the smell of you. From this first day

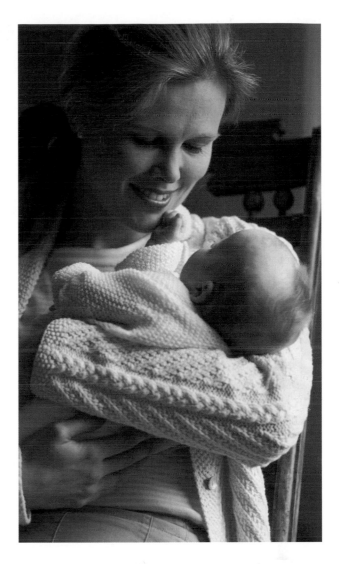

of life, you, with your partner, are everything to this newborn person: warmth, shelter, comfort and security. It will take time for you all to be completely bonded to one another, but this will come.

## HOLDING AND HANDLING

Many new parents are frightened of handling a fragile tiny newborn, but there is nothing to be afraid of, as long as you hold him or her safely and confidently – babies quickly detect if the person holding them is unsure of what they are doing and they feel more secure and more comfortable if they are handled with conviction.

Always lift your baby slowly and gently, avoiding any jerky movements. Make sure that your baby's head is properly supported at all times, as newborn babies cannot support their own heads for the first few weeks. Hold your baby close and bend right over when lifting, sliding one hand under their head, and the other under their lower back.

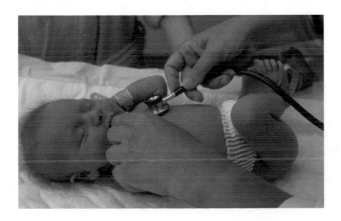

*Newborn babies are monitored by medical staff to ensure that all of their vital functions are working well.*

# Feeding your baby

All the nutrients your newborn baby receives come from milk. The options are to feed from the breast or from the bottle. Bottle-feeding is done either by using made-up 'formula milk' (that is, milk that is specially suited to babies) or by using milk expressed from your breasts (see page 136).

Experts agree that breastfeeding is the best way to nourish your baby. They recommend that, ideally, you should breastfeed for at least six months, although some women find that they are unable to feed their baby for this long. Other women are unable to breastfeed at all for a variety of reasons, including illness or inability to breastfeed successfully or easily, and there are also those who simply do not like the idea of breastfeeding. For these mothers, bottle-feeding with formula milk is the only answer, and even breastfeeding women may want to use bottles from time to time for reasons of convenience – when they are out and about, for example.

The commonest formula milk is cow's milk that has been modified to make it suitable. About one in ten infants is allergic to cow's milk formula. Soya and hydrolysate formula milks offer an alternative, but they have less in common with human milk than cow's milk does. So, if you can persevere with breastfeeding, your baby will benefit.

Ultimately, how you feed your baby is a very personal decision. Talk through your feelings with nursing staff, who will be happy to advise you. They will give you plenty of help with feeding issues but in the end you have to decide what is best for you and your baby.

## BREASTFEEDING

There are many advantages to breastfeeding, and paediatricians agree that it has the following benefits:
- Breast milk gives the baby protection from bugs, disease and allergy, such as eczema and asthma.
- Breastfed babies are less susceptible to stomach upsets and constipation.
- Breastfeeding helps to encourage the baby's facial development. It may also be responsible for the lower incidence of dental problems later in the baby's life.
- Breastfed babies are less likely to become overweight or obese later in life.
- Breastfeeding gives the newborn baby everything he or she needs and wants – physical contact with the mother, warmth and food. A crying baby usually finds breastfeeding more soothing and reassuring than bottle-feeding and is more easily consoled.

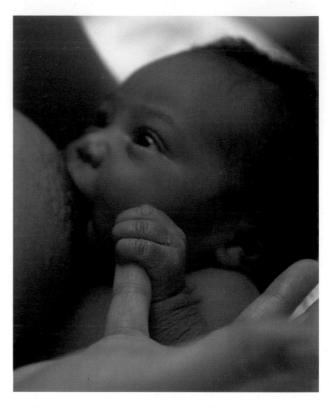

*Breastfeeding is a skill that may need to be learned. Once you get the hang of it, feeding your baby becomes a pleasurable experience for you both.*

- Breast milk is naturally sterile and the correct temperature – so mothers do not have the bother of making sure that bottle-feeding equipment is sterile and that the temperature of the milk is safe.
- Breastfeeding helps new mothers to get their figure back. Breastfeeding causes the release of a hormone, called oxytocin, which helps shrink the uterus.
- Breastfeeding reduces a woman's risk of developing breast cancer in later life.

### What breast milk contains

Human breast milk contains all the nutrients your baby needs, in the right proportions. It has:
- Enough water to quench the baby's thirst.
- Protein for body building.
- Fat for energy and growth.
- Carbohydrate, in the form of lactose, for energy.
- Vitamins and minerals.
- Antibodies and iron-binding protein, which make the baby's intestine less vulnerable to bacteria and protect against a number of serious illnesses.

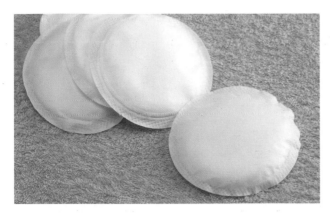

*Breast pads, tucked inside your bra, are the answer to leaking breasts, which can be an embarrassment and may also lead to sore, cracked nipples. Both disposable and washable pads are available.*

At the beginning of a feed, the baby gets foremilk, which has a high water content. When he or she continues to suck, the hindmilk comes: this is rich in calories and helps the baby to grow. You should therefore let the baby feed from one breast for as long as he or she wishes.

### Getting used to breastfeeding

Breastfeeding can be difficult at the start – it doesn't always come naturally to the baby or the mother. It may take as long as a fortnight to establish breastfeeding and another month or so for a pattern to develop. It is important to accept that there will be no routine at first. Your family doctor or the hospital can arrange for you to see a specialist breastfeeding counsellor or midwife.

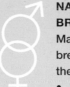

### NATURAL SOLUTIONS TO BREASTFEEDING PROBLEMS

Many women experience problems with breastfeeding at some stage. Natural therapies can offer some gentle solutions.

- To increase the production of breast milk, try herbal teas, such as raspberry leaves, goat's rue, fennel, dill, borage, nettle, vervain or cinnamon. Do not drink more than three cups a day.
- If you are finding breastfeeding difficult, homeopathic remedies may help. Suitable remedies may include bryonia, phytolacca, conium and belladonna, but see a homeopath for advice.
- Cracked nipples may be relieved by the homeopathic remedy castor equi 30C. Applying calendula cream can help, but wash it off completely before feeding.
- Ease the discomfort of engorged breasts by placing savoy cabbage leaves directly on them (an ice-cold flannel or a bag of frozen vegetables wrapped in a flannel are other options).

Talk to your doctor or health visitor if you have any anxieties about your feeding technique or milk supply, or if you experience symptoms such as fever or swelling or redness of the breast.

## How to get your baby latched on

Hold your baby in a position that will be comfortable, relaxed and secure – you may like to prop your arm on a cushion. Place your baby so that his or her body forms a straight line from your breast. That way, the baby's head doesn't have to turn in order to feed. Make sure that the baby is held high enough to reach your nipple easily.

The important thing is to get your baby 'latched on' (fixed on) to the breast properly. This will help to make sure your baby gets a good milk supply. It will also minimize problems such as breasts that are engorged with milk (because the milk is not flowing well) and nipple soreness.

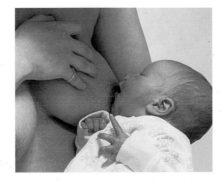

**1** The baby's mouth should be wide open before you present your breast for feeding. Bring your nipple close to his or her nose, and let the baby take it into the mouth. However, the nipple should be entirely within the baby's mouth and his or her jaws clamped on to your breast rather than on to the nipple itself.

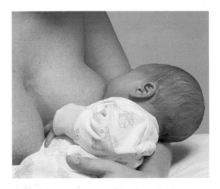

**2** Let the baby feed at one breast for as long as he or she wants. Then offer the other breast. If the baby doesn't want to continue feeding, offer this breast first next time around. Don't worry about having no idea when to stop – a baby will usually let you know when he or she has had enough milk.

### Breastfeeding in the first few days

Tension is probably the biggest cause of initial breastfeeding problems, so try to relax and enjoy your baby as much as possible. Your breasts do not start to make milk until they are stimulated by a complex hormonal reaction that takes place after the birth. Before this happens, the breasts produce colostrum, a creamy, yellowish substance which you may have noticed leaking during the last few months of pregnancy.

In the first few days of your baby's life, you are feeding him or her colostrum. This gives valuable protection from bacterial infections and illnesses the mother has had in the past or has been immunized against. It cannot be artificially reproduced.

### Expressing breast milk

There may be times when you would like the convenience of feeding your baby from a bottle, but you would still like to use your own milk. You may also be having problems with breastfeeding due to engorged breasts.

You can express milk from your breasts either by hand, or with a manual pump (see page 112), the latter method being much faster and easier. Always wash your hands before expressing milk, and make sure that any equipment is sterilized. With a manual pump, you simply fit the funnel over the areola of the breast so that it forms a good, tight seal. You then use a plunger or lever to express the milk. Expressed milk should be kept in a bottle with a tight-fitting lid and refrigerated until needed. Store it for up to a couple of days in a refrigerator, or for up to six months or so in a freezer.

### BOTTLE-FEEDING

Many women find this more convenient than breastfeeding and bottle-feeding with formula milk is a good way of nourishing babies whose mothers cannot breastfeed. Formula milk can be made up from powders that are basically dried milk or can be bought in liquid form, the latter being more expensive. Other options include various organic formula products and soya products, for babies with a cow's milk allergy. Feeding your baby with formula milk can be more time-consuming than breastfeeding and does not have the same health benefits. However, there are various advantages to this method:

- Anyone can feed the baby, not just you. Your partner can share the feeding, which may help bonding between baby and father.
- If you need to return to work, bottle-feeding can be more convenient. It means that you can go out without the baby for longer periods.
- Bottle-feeding may be useful if you are recovering from a Caesarean or difficult delivery and if you are ill. It is also good for premature or sick babies who are too weak to suck.

### What formula milk contains

- Water, but not enough, so your baby will need extra drinks of boiled water.
- Protein, but in too high a concentration, so it has to be diluted. This process lowers the calorie content of the feed, which is supplemented by lactose.
- Fat, which is less easily absorbed than breastmilk fat.
- Carbohydrate, but in insufficient quantity, so lactose has to be added.
- Vitamins and minerals, but not in the right amounts, so many formulas are enriched with extra vitamins and extra iron.

### BURPING YOUR BABY

The aim of burping your baby – rubbing or patting his or her back – is to bring up any air that your baby may have swallowed during feeding, as trapped air can cause a baby some discomfort.

Trapped air is more common when babies are fed from a bottle because there is more opportunity for air to enter the baby's mouth. When babies are breastfeeding, their mouths are usually so closely locked onto the breast that little air can get in.

The two basic ways to burp babies are to sit them on your lap so that they are leaning forwards (they shouldn't bend at the waist) and are supported securely round their chest. Now pat gently on the back. Do not pat too firmly – this may make your baby regurgitate their feed. Another method is to hold your baby against your shoulder and rub their back gently, using upward strokes. Make sure that you have an old towel over your shoulder in case your baby brings up a little milk (known as possetting). Don't worry that there is something wrong if your baby does not burp – it simply means he or she had no need to do so.

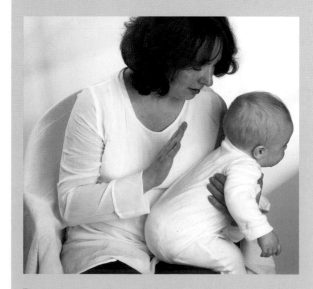

*Do not pat or rub too hard – go gently.*

### Preparing dried formula feeds

You should find clear instructions on the can or packet, and you must follow these carefully. Never add more powder than instructed in the hope of making the feed more nourishing, as this will give your baby too little water and too much protein and fat. Equally, don't add too little powder or the feed will not be nourishing enough. The water that you mix with the powder feed must be water that has been freshly boiled and allowed to cool slightly. Measure the water after it has boiled and cooled; if you do so before then you risk using too little water as you will have lost some through evaporation.

## KEEPING CLEAN

All equipment associated with feeding must be kept thoroughly clean or sterilized, in order to reduce the risk of your baby catching any gastro-intestinal infection – newborns are very susceptible to such infections. Make sure that you always wash your hands before touching feeding equipment and giving the bottle to your baby. Also, always keep bottles of prepared formula feed in the refrigerator, but never for longer than 24 hours – prepare at the time if at all possible.

Methods of cleaning equipment are: placing in boiling water for at least five minutes (allow to cool before using); using a sterilizing tank and chemicals; using a steamer; using a microwave sterilizer. Before sterilizing equipment, wash the equipment in warm soapy water or a dishwasher. Make sure that everything is properly rinsed, and that teats are especially well cleaned.

When using a sterilizing tank, fill the tank half full with cold water and add a sterilizing tablet. When the tablet has dissolved, put in your equipment. Fill the bottles with water to keep them under the water and then fill the tank up with cold water.

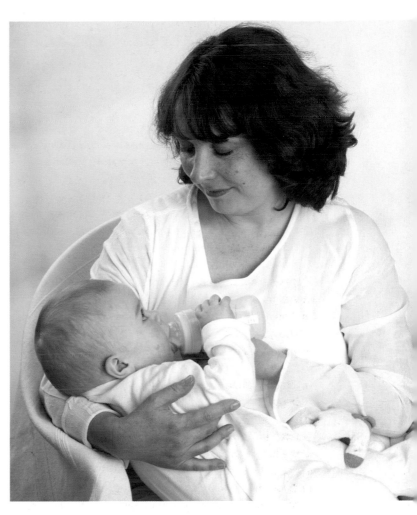

*A bottle-fed baby must be well supported at a slight angle with the head raised, so they can swallow and breathe easily without choking. Warm a bottle of formula milk in a bowl of warm water (not a microwave), splash a few drops on your inner wrist to see if it is tepid and unscrew the teat ring a little so the teat won't close up.*

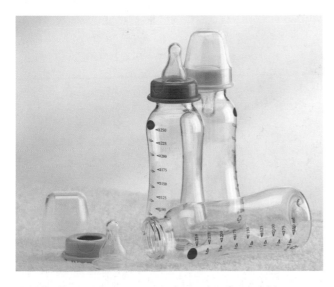

*Any bottles and teats must always be thoroughly sterilized to reduce the risk of infection.*

### CLEANING BOTTLES AND TEATS

Using warm, soapy water, clean inside the bottle very thoroughly with a brush and then rub the teats. Many of the bottle-cleaning brushes available now have a special teat-cleaner on the end of the handle.

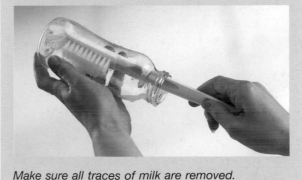

*Make sure all traces of milk are removed.*

# Changing and bathing

Parents are often daunted by the idea of changing and bathing a baby, but if you are patient and allow yourself some trial and error, you should have few problems.

## NAPPIES

There has never been such a wide range of nappy (diaper) options, so every parent can find something to suit:

- Disposables. Choose eco-friendly disposables rather than ordinary, standard types. Standard ones contain chemicals, especially in the absorbant gels used, that it is thought could be harmful to a baby. Disposal of these nappies causes problems for the environment.
- Fabric nappies. These reusable nappies are sold in a vast range of forms, from the classic terry towelling square to ready-shaped fabric nappies that close with integral fasteners (such as poppers) or with separate plastic fasteners (the modern equivalent of nappy pins). Many fabric nappies can be adjusted to fit a growing baby and you can use laundering services to clean them – such services tend to favour 'pre-folded' fabric nappies, now widely available.
- Liners. These fit right inside a fabric nappy to catch waste. Disposable liners that you simply flush away are very popular, and biodegradeable types are available. You can also buy washable fabric ones, which can be reused.
- Wraps and pants. These are reusable and fit over the top of nappies. The most natural option is a cotton wrap, with an inner waterproof layer, that closes with poppers or Velcro-type fastenings.
- All-in-ones. These are typically a cotton inner nappy permanently attached to a waterproof cover and fastened with poppers. The whole thing can be machine-washed and tumble-dried. These take some time to dry and seem costly as an initial outlay.

## CHANGING AND CLEANING

Always check for redness or rashes. Nappy rash is common but quickly treated – try soothing calendula cream and homeopathic calendula powder. Never use talc on your baby (or on yourself), even unperfumed kinds, as it has been linked with possible harmful effects. Wash the baby often and change the nappy as often as necessary. Allow the baby to be without a nappy for short intervals each day, so that air can circulate – warm, damp areas can lead to rashes.

To clean your baby before putting on a new nappy, use cotton wool with lots of warm water or just a gentle, non-perfumed lotion (especially if he or she has a rash). Avoid soaps if possible, especially perfumed and coloured ones, and try to steer clear of disposable wipes, which strip skin of natural oils. Clean girls from front to back, to avoid spreading germs into the vagina or urethra. Do not separate the labia or clean inside. When cleaning a boy's penis and testicles, do not pull back the foreskin. Dry by patting gently, right into the folds, with a soft towel.

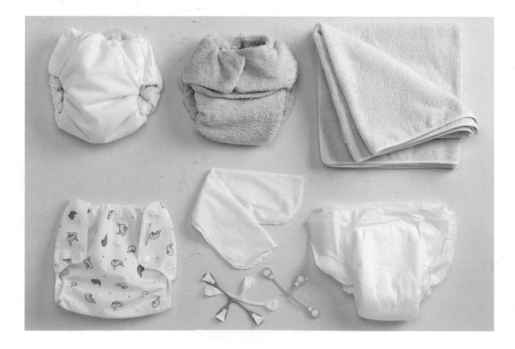

*Top row, from left: all-in-one washable nappy (diaper) with integral pants, shaped fabric nappy, terry squares. Bottom row from left: washable waterproof over-pants, washable fabric nappy liner and plastic fasteners for some fabric nappies (instead of safety pins), biodegradeable disposable nappy. The Internet is a great source of companies offering natural, eco-friendly options.*

# Changing a terry nappy

The simplest type of fabric nappy (diaper) is the old-fashioned terry towelling square, which you will need to fold and fix to form a nappy yourself. The method shown is the 'kite' method, although there are many others.

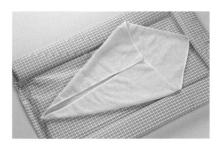

**1** Open up the square. Fold the sides in as shown (overlap these for a newborn, for extra absorbancy).

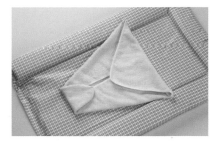

**2** Now fold down the top edge and fold up the bottom edge, leaving a space in between.

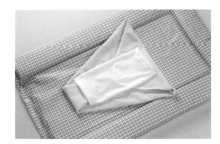

**3** Place a liner on top – either the disposable kind or a washable and reusable one (the latter is seen here).

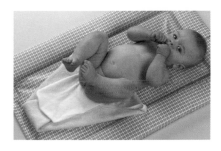

**4** Position your baby on top of the nappy. His or her waist should be aligned with the top edge of the folded square.

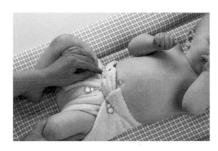

**5** Bring the sides in and the bottom part up between the legs. Tuck the central panel into the corners of the side pieces. Fix with a modern 'pin'.

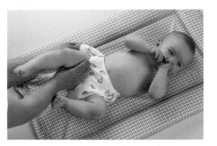

**6** Now put a waterproof wrap or pants over the top of the nappy, to stop your baby from staining his or her clothes.

## BATHING YOUR BABY

This is a good way to hold your baby in the bath, until he or she is able to sit up and play. Never leave a baby unattended in the bath – even for a minute and even if he or she is in a bath seat. Always check the temperature of the water before placing the baby in it. Do not let anyone who is not familiar with bathing children do this for you unless you are there, too.

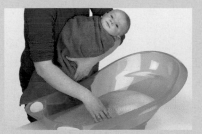

**1** Cradle the baby in your left arm as you test the temperature. (Use your right arm if left-handed.)

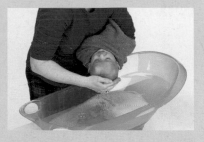

**2** Support the baby's back, neck and head as you wash the hair with your right hand.

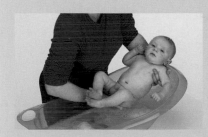

**3** Hold under the left arm and bottom and lower the baby into the bath.

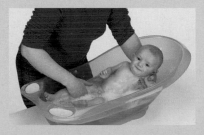

**4** Continue holding under the arm as you wash with your right hand.

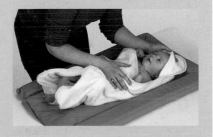

**5** Lift the baby out. Wrap the head and body in a towel, and dry well.

# Coping with the early days

If you had your baby in hospital, you may stay in the maternity unit for anything between six hours to three days, and even up to ten days if there have been complications. When you get home, it may feel good to relax in your own environment once again. However, most women also feel overwhelmed at this point – partly due to the action of your hormones and partly because you are adjusting to the unfamiliar experience of being a parent. Mothers with older children are likely to experience this feeling too, and they may feel exhausted at the prospect of dealing with everybody's needs. These first weeks can be a demanding time. It may be reassuring to know that things settle down after about three months or so, but that can seem like a very long time.

Seek advice from your community midwife, health visitor or doctor if anything bothers you and make time to discuss things supportively with your partner. In the meantime, eat well (foods that are rich in vitamins B2 and B6, zinc and magnesium may help to normalize hormone levels), and try to get some fresh air every day – if possible, have a short walk with your partner and the baby so that you can enjoy being a family together.

### RECOVERING FROM THE BIRTH

You may have to cope with various discomforts after the birth. If you have had an episiotomy or you have torn, your body will need time to heal. It may be helpful to take the homeopathic remedy arnica if there is any bruising but do not apply anything to the actual cut and sutures. Bathe

> **❝** You are likely to be unusually emotional. Give yourself time to get back to normal. **❞**

the area twice a day and dry with a warm (not hot) hairdryer since wetness will impede the healing process. If you have painful haemorrhoids, see your doctor. Eat plenty of high-fibre foods and apply a cold compress or soothing over-the-counter cream.

You are likely to be unusually emotional and fatigue will be a problem. Give yourself time to get back to normal and get plenty of rest. Try not to do too much, other than care for your baby – and let other people help out.

### THE BABY BLUES

Most women experience the baby blues, in which they feel weepy for no obvious reason and experience a sense of helplessness. This usually happens around the fifth day after the delivery. If you feel awful, let someone know – your partner, a nurse, a doctor or whoever you find most approachable. These feelings will pass.

### POSTNATAL DEPRESSION

A spell of the baby blues is normal for new mothers, and doesn't last long. It must not be confused with postnatal depression, however. Postnatal depression tends to occur later than baby blues, and the symptoms are those of classic depression. The mother may feel misery, fear and anger – directed at herself, her partner, her baby, or anyone else around her. Irritability, fatigue and sleeplessness are the hallmarks. The depression may not show itself until some months after the birth. Symptoms can include:

• Losing one's zest for life.
• Difficulty in sleeping.
• Waking early in the morning.
• Changes in appetite – eating more or less than usual.
• General feelings of apathy.
• Finding it hard to concentrate.
• Uncontrollable thoughts.
• Despair or suicidal feelings.

*Yoga may be very beneficial in the early months after birth to get you back in shape and help you cope with the demands of parenthood. As the baby grows older, he or she will enjoy practising with you. Ask your doctor when he or she advises that you should start exercising.*

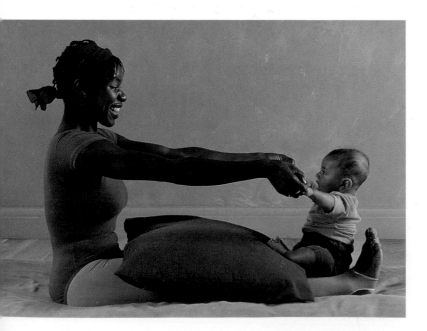

Postnatal depression can be very debilitating. At its worst, the mother may harm herself or the baby. Immediate professional help, via the family doctor or the health visitor, is therefore very important if depression is making it difficult for you to function, or if you are having harmful thoughts about yourself or your baby. You will not be judged: depression is an illness and your doctor can help you to cope and to get better.

Women with mild depression may experience a sense of apathy or misery, as well as early-morning wakefulness or other symptoms. It is still important that you tell your health visitor or doctor about how you are feeling. Natural therapies such as acupuncture, aromatherapy or cranial osteopathy can often help to alleviate some of the symptoms of depression.

Simple tasks can feel overwhelming if you are suffering from depression. Ask your partner, friends or relatives for extra support – help with housework, for example.

## SLEEP PATTERNS

The biggest problem for new parents is often lack of sleep – it is hard to function if you are deprived of rest. Understanding your baby's sleep may help you and your partner cope with interrupted nights. A newborn baby is awake for six to eight hours out of every 24, often for an hour or more at a time. Some babies are more wakeful

*It is unlikely that your baby will feel sleepy when you do. This means that most parents need to devise a sleeping schedule that includes daytime naps.*

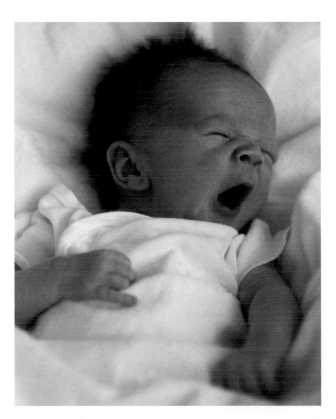

than others, The duration of sleep depends on a child's age and personality, the need for food, and also on the length of his or her daytime rests. At first, babies rarely sleep for longer than three to five hours at a time. However, by the age of four months most babies will sleep for six to ten hours at a time. They can also stay awake for several hours. Premature babies usually sleep for more than 16 hours per day, but within a year their sleep requirement will match that of full-term babies.

The main difficulty is that a baby's sleep patterns usually won't coincide with yours. Most adults like to sleep for about seven to nine hours every night, but a baby may wake up at 1 a.m. and then stay awake until just before dawn. Alternatively, the baby may sleep right through until 4 a.m. and then not sleep again for the remainder of the night. The only way to cope with this is to take extra naps in the day, and try to remain as calm as possible.

A baby needs to sleep in order to grow and mature. If your baby is tired but not sleepy, there are ways you can help him or her to drop off. Carrying a baby around in a sling may lull him or her to sleep – babies derive a sense of security from physical proximity and warmth. Rocking the baby and singing or playing music to him or her may also help. Some parents find that babies like 'white-noise' sounds such as that of a vacuum cleaner: you could try recording these sounds and playing it quietly if the baby won't settle.

# Checklist of common problems

Some of the most common problems your baby may develop are dealt with below. Contact your health visitor or doctor if you have any worries about your baby's health. Note that the essential oil remedies mentioned should ideally only be used for babies over about two to three months old, as essential oils are very concentrated.

**Crying** Babies cry for many different reasons:

- Tiredness.
- Hunger.
- Need for physical reassurance.
- Boredom.
- Being too cold.
- Being too warm.
- Feeling uncomfortable (tight clothing etc).
- A full nappy (diaper).
- Being ill or in pain.

Make sure that the baby's obvious needs are catered for first. If the baby continues to cry after being fed and changed, try some of these: rocking the baby rhythmically, patting, stroking, caressing and smiling at him or her. You could also try soothing baby massage. If your baby cries a lot, try adding a herbal infusion to the baby's bath, such as chamomile, hops, lavender or lemon balm. Before you put him or her to bed, massage the feet and limbs with any of these herbal oils. You may wish to take him or her to a cranial osteopath (see page 145), particularly if the delivery was difficult. Sound sometimes solves the problem, so try playing music, singing to your baby, or playing a musical instrument yourself.

It is unwise to ignore a crying baby, however trying the constant crying may become. If you start to feel that you are at the end of your tether, put the baby in her cot or pram and telephone your health visitor, a relative or a friend to talk. Ask for help if you need it.

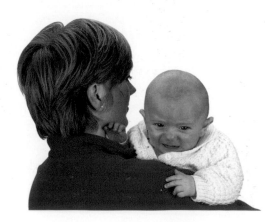

**Colic** Some babies experience bouts of painful intestinal cramp (colic), which usually occur from within a few days of birth up until about three months. The baby will howl, maybe for hours on end, drawing the knees up over the stomach. Colic typically occurs during the evening, with the baby being quite contented and well during the day. Be sure to feed the baby as slowly as possible. It may also help to give an aromatherapy massage using 1 drop Roman chamomile oil diluted in 150ml (5fl oz) almond oil towards the end of each afternoon. Fennel is the traditional herbal remedy for colic: before you feed the baby, try giving her a 25ml (1½ tbsp) infusion: add 1.5-2.5ml (¼-½ tsp) of the crushed herb to 100ml (7 tbsp) boiling water, leave for a few minutes, then strain. You can add the leftover infusion to the baby's bath. Homeopathic remedies include pulsatilla, nux vomica, aconite, dulcamara and bryonia, but seek the advice of a qualified homeopath.

**Cradle cap** A thick circle of dead skin may form on the scalp of a newborn baby. This will eventually clear up of its own accord. However, you can soften the scales so that they drop off more easily by using a massage oil such as almond, or blend 1 drop rose and 1 drop chamomile essential oil to 30ml (2 tbsp) almond oil. Massage very gently into the scalp for one to two days just before bedtime. The following morning shampoo with a natural baby shampoo and rinse with 7.5ml (1½ tsp) cider vinegar added to the water. Do not try to pick off the scales, as this can lead to infection.

**Nappy rash** One of the best ways to prevent nappy (diaper) rash is to allow the baby to be without a nappy as often as possible. You may also like to add one to two drops of chamomile or lavender oil, well-diluted in whole milk, to the baby's bath water. Jojoba oil is excellent for treating nappy rash: it leaves a fine waxy coating on the baby's skin, which moisturizes and soothes. Apply a little of the following blend when you change the nappy: 1 drop lavender and 1 drop rose or Roman chamomile to 30ml (2 tbsp) jojoba carrier oil. If the skin is very sore, use 10 per cent calendula (marigold) carrier oil in the blend. The homeopathic options include calendula or Rescue Remedy cream.

*If your baby is colicky and cries for long periods, try to give yourself regular periods away from the house. Call on friends and relatives to help.*

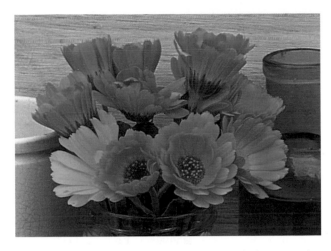

*Calendula cream is very healing and may help to soothe the soreness of nappy rash. It is available from large pharmacists or health-food stores.*

**Colds and flu** If your baby is sniffling or appears unwell, take his or her temperature. If it is raised, consult your family doctor without delay. If the temperature exceeds 38.5°C (101°F), seek emergency medical assistance. For mild symptoms, a warm, humid atmosphere loosens catarrh, while squirting a little breast milk into a baby's nostrils helps to dry the passages out.

**Cough** Again, a warm, humid atmosphere can help. If your baby's cough persists for more than a day or seems severe, seek immediate medical treatment.

**Croup** Croup often starts with the baby losing his or her voice and with the breathing sounding hoarse or croaky. This can lead to croup, which is characterized by spasms of coughing and difficulty in breathing. Croup sounds are not unlike the bark made by a sea lion. If your baby suffers from croup, try to relieve his or her breathing with steam. Boil a kettle and remove the lid so that the steam wafts over the baby. Light a vaporizer in the bedroom half an hour before baby's bedtime (any large pharmacy can supply one), with eucalyptus oil added for slightly older babies. Central heating should be kept as low as possible and the window should be open a little so that the air is less dry. If your baby's breathing continues to be laboured, speak to your family doctor (croup can sometimes be confused with whooping cough). If the breathing rapidly becomes worse, seek emergency medical treatment.

**Diarrhoea and vomiting** The main danger here is dehydration. Diarrhoea (in which the faeces are more liquid and frequent than normal) is not uncommon and may have various causes. As for vomiting, it is quite normal for babies to be sick after eating. If the vomiting or diarrhoea is mild and clears quickly, then help counteract

the conditions as follows: breastfed babies should be given short, very regular feeds, while bottle-fed babies will benefit from plenty of sips of plain, boiled and cooled water. If either condition persists, or is accompanied by other symptoms such as fever, then seek immediate medical treatment.

**Constipation** If your baby becomes constipated (straining but unable to pass stools), offer extra fluid. If bottle-feeding, ensure that you are making formulas up correctly. If the condition does not pass very quickly or other symptoms appear, then seek medical help.

**Eye infection** Bathe the eyes in cooled, boiled water, using a separate piece of clean cotton wool or tissue for each eye and wiping from the inner corner to the outer one (having washed your hands first). Breast milk can also be used, as it is anti-bacterial. Unless the condition is very mild and disappears rapidly, you should consult your health visitor or your family doctor.

**DANGER SYMPTOMS**

Seek emergency medical treatment if your baby or child exhibits any of these:
- Breathlessness or difficulty in breathing.
- Unexplained, abnormal drowsiness.
- Fever of 38.5°C (101°F) or more.
- Convulsions (fits).
- Any severe pain or obvious distress.
- Repeated or persistent vomiting, diarrhoea or constipation.
- Refusing food.
- Stiff neck, especially if combined with dislike of bright light.
- Severe headache.
- Impaired vision, especially with headache.

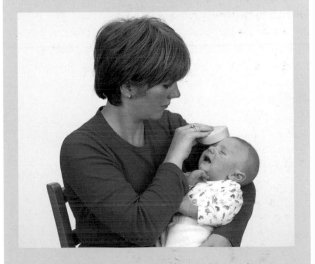

*If a baby is hot, sponge the face with cool water.*

# Common Qs and As

**Q**: My nipples don't stick out and I can't see how my baby will be able to feed. Is there anything that I can do?

**A**: You will probably be fine. Health professionals used to recommend the use of nipple shields for inturned nipples. However, they rarely do nowadays because they know that the nipple is likely to become more defined once the milk comes in.

Usually the let-down reflex, which allows milk to be expressed from the breast, assists in the nipple becoming more prominent. Otherwise, you may find it helpful to splash very cold water over the breast, or even hold ice cubes against it for a minute or two, to help the nipple out.

**Q**: My bust is tiny (30 AA). Will I be able to make enough milk for my baby?

**A**: Don't worry – the size of the breast is not relevant, and you almost certainly will be able to feed your baby. Start off by feeding every two hours or so, as this helps to establish a good flow.

Many women believe that they are not making enough milk to meet their baby's needs, and this is often the reason for a specialist hospital referral. However, paediatricians often find that the baby is thriving, and weight checks show that weight gain is on course. The only problem is that the mother thinks she is not providing enough milk.

Rest assured that you will soon know about it if your baby feels hungry or undernourished. Talk to your midwife if you think that this is the case.

**Q**: My breasts become engorged at the wrong time. When they are full, my baby doesn't seem that interested in feeding. Then, when she is hungry, there doesn't seem to be enough to satisfy her. What is going on?

**A**: This does happen in the early days while you and the baby are getting used to one another. It may take as long as several weeks for a harmonious pattern to develop. So, do not despair.

Ask your family doctor, community midwife or health visitor for an appointment to see a breastfeeding counsellor if the situation continues. Difficulties in breastfeeding are often a problem of technique – the mother's or the baby's.

**Q**: I had a very difficult birth and wasn't able to breastfeed or hold my baby for the first few weeks. You hear so much about the importance of bonding in the first days, and I feel I have failed her. How can I make it up to her?

**A**: There is no need to feel that you have failed your baby in any way. There have obviously been very good reasons why you and your baby were unable to be together for the first few weeks of her life. This often happens with premature babies and with ill babies, when the baby is whisked away to an intensive baby care unit, usually at a central teaching hospital, while the mother is left in the local hospital where she delivered.

As for making it up to her, smiles, cuddles, laughing and feeding – and even changing her nappies with love and care – will all help to bring about the bonding process. Your baby will not remember the first few weeks, but she will respond to all your love now. Just be positive and enjoy her.

**Q**: **How does everyone else cope with fatigue? I feel as if I am sleepwalking.**

**A**: The best advice is to take each day as it comes. When you are really tired, you just have to go with the flow. Take every opportunity you can to sleep, and if you can't sleep, rest.

Make as few plans as possible, and don't worry if you do not achieve something that you set out to do. If you have the option, don't go back to work until you feel on top of things.

**Q**: **My newborn baby is often sick when he is in the car. How can I prevent this?**

**A**: First of all, consider whether you are rushing to get out of the house. If so, slow down. Be sure that you leave home in a calm and unflurried state with plenty of time to allow you to reach your destination. This helps to reduce anxiety in you, which would readily transmit itself to your baby.

Feed your baby at least an hour before you want to take him or her out in the car. It is also worth considering whether your baby has had enough sleep when they first get in the car – take him or her out for a trial run when you know they are rested.

How smoothly you drive and at what speed will have a bearing on how well your baby travels. Keep your speed down, avoid jerky manoeuvres and don't attempt to overtake.

If the problem continues, there are herbal and homeopathic options with which to treat carsickness. However, it is much better to try to treat the cause rather than the symptoms, particularly since your baby is so young.

**Q**: **We have both a dog and a cat. Should we be worried about having them around a newborn baby?**

**A**: Be very careful and take no risks. Dogs do suffer from jealousy, and have been known to attack with absolutely no warning. Cats may also react unpredictably. Do not leave your baby alone with the dog or cat, and keep the door to your baby's room shut while she is sleeping. Basically, if a pet shows signs of undue aggression towards others, then it may be a problem. If you are at all worried about either pet's behaviour, then regrettably the safest course of action would be to re-home him or her.

**Q**: **Quite a few of my friends and some of the other women in my antenatal group have taken their new babies to see a cranial osteopath. What is this?**

**A**: Some people take their newborn baby to a cranial osteopath to check and treat any birth trauma, especially to the head and neck. Treatment consists of the practitioner placing his or her hands on the baby's body and identifying any areas of restriction or tension. Gentle stroking is used to release these. It can be a very effective therapy for babies, particularly in treating sleeping problems.

Cranial osteopathy is a branch of osteopathy, and so practitioners have been through rigorous training. Be sure that anyone you take your baby to see is suitably qualified and experienced in dealing with young babies.

# CHAPTER SIX
## Natural therapies

" Natural therapies can provide a really positive cornerstone to your pregnancy care programme. "

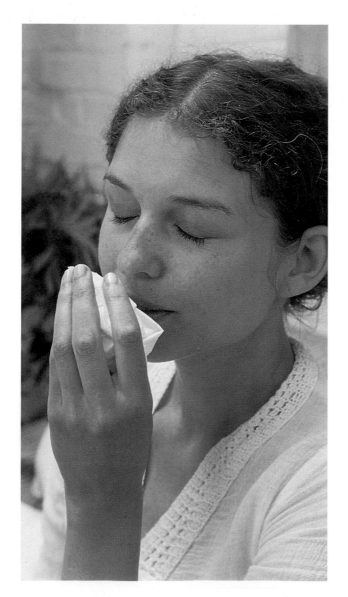

The aim of this chapter is to give some valuable background to, and additional information on, the various natural therapies that are mentioned throughout the main body of the book.

The many natural therapies that are now available can provide a really positive cornerstone to any woman's pregnancy care programme. While there is a wide range of opinion about the type and degree of physical benefit brought by therapies such as herbalism and homeopathy, few would deny that such therapies can provide enormous support throughout the emotional highs and lows that are commonly experienced by most pregnant women and new mothers (and also fathers). As for the physical aspect, it seems simple common sense to accept that anything which promotes a healthier body will help to ease the path to a better pregnancy and an easier birth and will also help to prepare both parents for the considerable demands of looking after a newborn baby.

*The benefits of aromatherapy can be enjoyed in many different ways, from adding oils to your bath to sniffing a few drops on a handkerchief.*

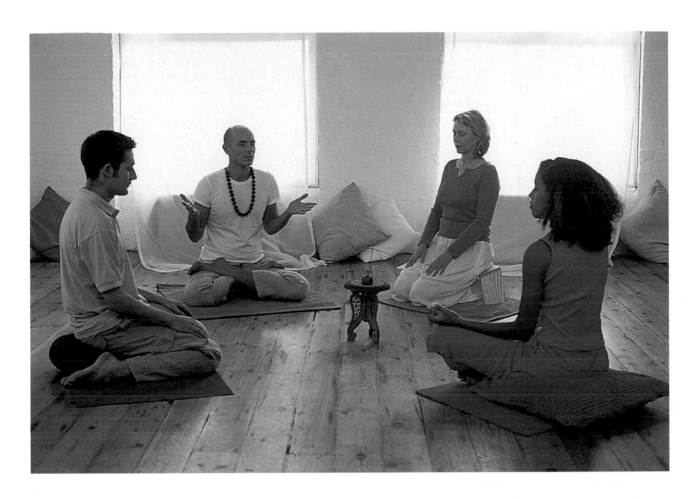

Natural remedies may alleviate ailments in pregnancy and speed recovery after the birth. However, they should be used with caution: many therapies need to be adapted for pregnant women, and others are not suitable in the first weeks. It cannot be stated enough that it is always important to seek out a qualified practitioner who is used to working with pregnant women. Tell the therapist if you are pregnant (or if you are trying to conceive). Ask your doctor about any therapy you are planning to try and tell him or her about any that you are receiving, and also about any recommendations that therapists have made to you. Be careful, but do enjoy yourself and pick a therapy that suits you – that way you will be sure to stick with it.

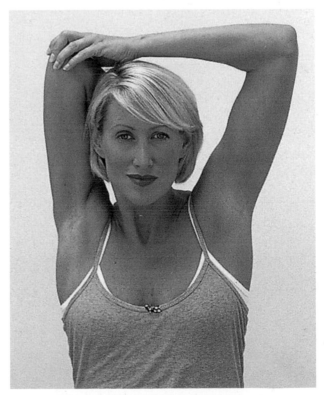

*Top: Meditation can bring much-needed mental stillness at this challenging time. You may want to enjoy it as a couple by joining a group class.*

*Regular yoga and simple stretching exercises help to improve breathing technique and pelvic flexibility as well as calming the mind and emotions.*

# Herbalism

Many plants have therapeutic properties, which can be used to improve health and treat illness. For the mother-to-be, herbs can offer support in all kinds of ways, from alleviating morning sickness to easing varicose veins.

Many modern pharmaceutical medicines are derived from plants, although science has made it possible to isolate active ingredients or recreate synthetic versions. By contrast, herbal remedies use parts of the whole plant – roots, seeds, petals or leaves. Herbalists say that the interaction of all the herb's ingredients promotes healing in a holistic (whole body) way rather than just attacking a single symptom or disease.

### HERBAL MEDICINE AND PREGNANCY

Although herbal medicines are usually gentler than chemical ones, they can have powerful effects. Many herbs should not be used in pregnancy and herbs should never be self-prescribed. A few herbs are gentle enough to be used in infusion form during pregnancy. In the first trimester, ginger tea may alleviate morning sickness and aid the digestion. Later on, dandelion, meadowsweet, lime flower and nettle can be helpful. Drink no more than three cups of herbal tea a day. Herbal ointments, compresses and poultices can ease symptoms relating to pregnancy, birth and breastfeeding. For example, calendula cream is often recommended for cracked nipples.

Always see a qualified medical herbalist and tell them about any drugs that you are taking since they may interact badly with natural remedies; for the same reason, tell your doctor about any remedies you are taking. A medical herbalist should take a medical history, examine you and advise on diet and lifestyle as well as prescribing remedies.

### HERBS NOT TO USE IN PREGNANCY

- angelica
- barberry
- black cohosh
- bloodroot
- buckthorn
- celery
- cinchona
- cinnamon
- cottonroot
- feverfew
- golden seal
- greater celandine
- juniper
- liferoot
- male fern
- mandrake
- mistletoe
- mugwort
- nutmeg
- pennyroyal
- poke root
- rhubarb
- rosemary
- rue
- saffron
- sage
- southernwood
- tansy
- thuja
- thyme
- wormwood

# Homeopathy

This gentle therapy can help with many of the physical symptoms and difficult emotions experienced during pregnancy. The remedies are derived from natural substances, and aim to stimulate the body's capacity for healing.

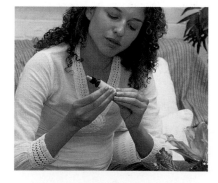

*Flower remedies are homeopathic remedies said to ease negative states of mind. Add a few drops to a glass of water and sip.*

Homeopathy is based on the idea that 'like cures like': so a substance that causes illness can also be used to cure it. The remedies have been so diluted that only a trace of the active ingredient remains. In this state, they are far too weak to cause harm, but homeopaths believe that the minute dose can promote self-healing and cure the very symptoms that it may cause if taken in large amounts. Homeopathic remedies are considered very safe in pregnancy. They can help to relieve many ailments, such as morning sickness, and to speed recovery after the birth. Self-help remedies are available from many pharmacies, but it is much better to consult a homeopath.

### SEEING A HOMEOPATH

A homeopath will take a full personal and medical history during the first session, which can last two hours. The homeopath needs to build up a picture of your habits and preferences as well as your mental, physical and emotional make-up. This information enables him or her to assess your 'constitutional type' and choose from the 2,000 remedies at their disposal. You may also be given advice about your diet and lifestyle.

See a homeopath who is experienced in treating pregnant women and contact them if any symptoms worsen (this may be part of the healing process). Note that peppermint, coffee and tea can nullify the effect, and you should avoid drinking or eating for 15 minutes after taking a remedy.

# Aromatherapy

Aromatherapists use aromatic oils from herbs and flowers. Certain oils have a wonderfully relaxing effect, others help to relieve conditions such as the indigestion that is common in pregnancy, or lift spirits during labour.

We do not know exactly how essential oils work, but it is thought that the scents trigger a reaction in smell receptors in the nostrils, which send messages to the brain. When the oils are used in massage, they also penetrate the skin and have a direct effect on the nerve endings here.

## BENEFITS OF AROMATHERAPY

In pregnancy, oils can be used to help the circulation, reducing the chance of varicose veins and haemorrhoids. Aromatherapy massage promotes skin elasticity and helps to prevent stretchmarks. Minor ailments such as constipation and heartburn may also be helped. Aromatherapy is well known for its relaxing effect, and a warm bath with a soothing oil such as Roman chamomile before bedtime can promote restful sleep. Mix four to six drops of essential oil with a carrier oil or whole milk, then add to a full bath (not to running water). Inhalation is another way of enjoying essential oils: put a few drops on a tissue or inhale steam from a bowl of hot water with some drops of oil added. Many oils cannot be used during pregnancy, as they may stimulate the uterus and cause miscarriage, so check first. It may be best to

**OILS TO AVOID IN PREGNANCY**

- basil
- cedarwood
- cinnamon bark
- clary sage
- cypress
- fennel
- hyssop
- juniper
- marjoram
- myrrh
- nutmeg
- oregano
- parsley
- peppermint
- rosemary
- sage
- savory
- thyme

avoid using essential oils entirely in the first trimester; see page 54 for good oils to use in the second trimester. Never apply essential oil directly to skin – always dilute it in a carrier: use one drop per 5ml (1 tsp) carrier; one drop per 10 ml (2 tsp) if pregnant. Do a patch test before use: apply diluted oil to a small area inside your wrist and wait 24 hours. If you have no reaction, the oil is safe. Women may be more sensitive when pregnant, so repeat a patch test at this time.

# Massage

Touch has been used to enhance health for thousands of years and is a powerful way of giving comfort and relieving pain. Massage is a leading touch therapy that can be especially helpful as a pain-relief tool in the delivery room.

The term 'massage' covers many different therapies. On the one hand, there is purely physical Western massage, which works on the muscles. On the other, there are forms of Eastern pressure massage, which seek to enhance energy flow along invisible pathways. These include shiatsu and acupressure. Massage also forms a vital element of therapies such as osteopathy, aromatherapy and reflexology.

## SWEDISH MASSAGE

In the West, most therapists practise Swedish massage. This system was devised by a Swedish gymnast, Per Henrik Ling, in the late 18th century. The techniques include:

- **Stroking** (effleurage) to relax. Firmer strokes are used to stimulate the circulation and release muscular tension.
- **Kneading** (petrissage) which relaxes tense muscles and increases blood flow to particular areas.
- **Friction** in which small, circular movements are made with the pads of the thumbs to break down areas of muscular spasm.

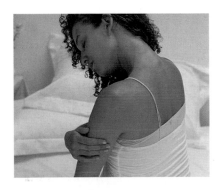

*Pleasurable touch on the skin encourages the release of endorphins (natural pain-killing chemicals), making massage a useful therapy in labour.*

- **Percussion** in which fast movements are made with the sides of the hands on fleshy areas. Avoid if pregnant.

In pregnancy, massage is good for backache and joint pain, and its relaxing effects mean it can help with depression, anxiety, blood pressure, digestive problems, headaches and insomnia. Stroking the lower back during labour can ease pain, but avoid deep pressure on the lower back or abdomen in pregnancy; never massage lumps, varicose veins or bruises.

# Acupuncture Practised for centuries in China, acupuncture is now widely available in the West, and can help with many pregnancy-related disorders.

Acupuncture is based on the idea that chi (energy) flows along invisible pathways – known as meridians – in the body. Illness and emotional upset occur when this energy flow is blocked. Fine needles are inserted into certain points on the meridians (this is swift and painless) to improve the

flow of chi and bring the body back to its natural state of equilibrium. Acupuncture is also used to treat specific complaints, such as back pain and digestion problems.

Acupuncture can relieve many pregnancy-related ailments, including morning sickness, constipation and poor circulation. It may also help with recurrent miscarriage. It is very important that you tell your practitioner that you are pregnant (or trying to conceive), since some points should not be stimulated in these cases.

Your practitioner will ask you many questions about, for example, your appetite, bowel movements, sleep and energy levels. Your pulses will be taken and your tongue checked. Your practitioner will also observe other details, such as the sound of your voice and the colour of your skin.

**OTHER ACUPUNCTURE TECHNIQUES**
Finger pressure (acupressure) can be used instead of needles to stimulate acupoints. This is less invasive than needling, and can be used for self-help. Another technique is moxibustion, where the herb moxa (mugwort) is burned on energy points.

# Shiatsu This term is Japanese for 'finger pressure'. Practitioners stimulate energy points linked with the vital organs to promote energy flow and better health.

Shiatsu practitioners use finger or hand pressure to encourage the flow of chi (energy) around the body. They may also use gentle stretching or rocking movements. Many Japanese people undergo regular shiatsu treatment. They believe that it can help to prevent illness as well as detect and treat any symptoms early on.

Shiatsu is a holistic system of healing, meaning that the whole person – mind, body and spirit – is treated at once. However, it can also be used to treat problems such as back pain, digestive problems, insomnia, depression,

migraine and toothache, and to help strengthen the immune system. Uses in pregnancy include dealing with backache and raised blood pressure, and pain-relief during labour.

Shiatsu should be kept simple and non-specific during the first three months of pregnancy, when all the baby's organ systems are developing. A practitioner can attend the birth to help with pain relief, or can teach the father or another birth assistant some simple pain-relief techniques with which to support the mother during her labour.

# Reflexology Reflexologists believe that every body part is linked by an energy pathway to a specific point on the foot.

In this pressure therapy, practitioners use finger pressure on the feet to detect and treat health problems. Reflexology is good for promoting general well-being and relaxation. A range of pregnancy-related problems can be tackled, from backache, digestive disorders and constipation to relieving pubic joint discomfort prior to the birth. Some midwives use the techniques to promote regular contractions and for pain relief during labour. One study found that reflexology could reduce a woman's need for pain relief, and cut the length of labour.

Reflexology should be used only after the first 12 weeks of pregnancy. Some areas – the heels, Achilles tendons and ankles – must be avoided as this can induce contractions.

A typical session begins with the reflexologist massaging your feet to relax them. After this, every area of your foot will be pressed and massaged in turn. Some areas may feel very sensitive – this is said to be a sign of imbalance. Tender points will receive extra massage in order to stimulate energy flow to the corresponding area of the body. This can sometimes be painful, but tenderness should ease as the massage continues. The reflexologist will adjust the pressure, depending on your sensitivity.

Your reflexologist may show you some techniques that you can practise at home. The hands also contain a 'map' of the body, and these are often recommended for self-help because they are easier to treat than the feet.

# Meditation This form of mental exercise can lead to greater inner

harmony, making it the ideal way to relax and deal with the stress of pregnancy.

Research has shown that regular meditation can reverse the effects of stress and help to alleviate ailments such as insomnia and digestive problems. Spending a few minutes each day in quiet contemplation can help women to cope with the challenges of pregnancy and new motherhood.

Practices vary but often involve concentrating on a single object, to still the mind. Common methods are to focus on your breathing or on an object such as a candle flame, or on a sound that you repeat many times (a mantra). Another technique is visualization, which involves picturing an object, a happy event or a beautiful scene in your mind's eye. In pregnancy, this may help anxiety and promote bonding. Imagine your baby developing healthy and strong, or prepare for the birth by imagining the birth canal opening.

**HYPNOTHERAPY**
This field has some general links with meditation practices. Hypnotherapists work by inducing a relaxed, trance-like state in their clients – a state in which clients are highly receptive to any suggestions, including suggestions for self-healing and relaxation.

Most people find it easier to learn in a group, while some prefer to practise meditation in conjunction with a practice based on physical movement, such as yoga or t'ai chi. Check with your doctor before starting if you have suffered from any form of psychiatric illness in the past. Sometimes meditation can bring up disturbing thoughts and images.

# Reiki Practitioners of this gentle hands-on therapy say that they act as

channels for the healing energy (ki/chi) that flows through the universe.

Reiki developed as a spiritual practice, but you do not have to subscribe to a particular philosophy to enjoy its benefits. Practitioners lay their hands on or just above a person's body, to direct energy wherever it is needed. Reiki may be helpful for minor ailments such as backache or constipation and many people find it deeply relaxing – it is often used for stress, anxiety and depression, including mild depression during and after pregnancy. Most doctors are sceptical, but see it as harmless so long as it is not used in place of medical treatment. It is safe in pregnancy.

In a typical session, the practitioner places his or her hands on different parts of your (fully clothed) body for several minutes at a time. Twelve basic positions are used: four on the head, four on the back and four on the front, relating to different energy centres in the body. You may feel a sensation of tingling or heat emanating from the practitioner's hands, said to be a sign of healing energy being drawn into your body. After a treatment, some people feel relaxed and sleepy; others feel energized. Anyone can set up as a teacher, so it is best to seek out reiki 'masters'.

# Colour therapy & crystal healing

Therapists say that colours and crystals give out vibrations that can improve well-being.

Colour therapists believe that colours transmit healing vibrations, and that these can be used to treat illness and improve well-being. Research has shown that colours can have a powerful effect on our mood. For example, blue can be very calming, while yellow can help to enhance learning ability. Therapists work in diferent ways. You may be asked to lie draped in coloured silks or to sit in front of a machine that directs coloured light at you.

If you visit a crystal healer, several crystals may be placed on different parts of your body – often over the body's energy centres (chakras) – to encourage healing. You may also be given a crystal to wear, carry or place in your home.

*Placing the crystal chrysocolla on the throat chakra promotes communication – vital for coping with pregnancy.*

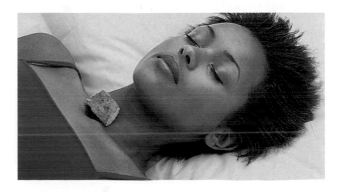

# Feng shui
The Chinese art of feng shui is based on the idea that a powerful life-force exists in everything in the universe and that buildings and rooms also contain this force.

Essentially, this is the art of arranging your home in order to harness positive energy, and using it to improve your health, relationships, career, fertility or other aspects of your life. One of the uses for parents-to-be is to create a harmonious nursery for their baby.

## DIFFERENT SCHOOLS OF THOUGHT
There are different approaches to feng shui. The traditional form incorporates Chinese astrology and the use of a special compass (the lo pan). Some practitioners use a tool called a bagua to determine which areas of your home relate to different aspects of your life. Many Western practitioners work intuitively, preferring to sense which areas of your home are lacking in chi (energy).

## SELF-HELP
Some aspects of feng shui can be used for self-help. However, much of the theory is complicated and using a practitioner is recommended if you want to ensure that your home is organized according to feng shui principles. It is a good idea to talk to a practitioner on the telephone before arranging a consultation. As with any complementary therapy, choose someone you feel comfortable with.

### DOES IT WORK?
Feng shui experts believe that your environment is only one of several influences on your life – your birth date, birth place and personal character are others. There is no proof that feng shui works, but it is widely practised in China and it does include common-sense ideas that will enhance the atmosphere of your home.

## WHAT A CONSULTATION INVOLVES
A feng shui practitioner will usually visit your home, but some practitioners work by post, using a floor plan. You should mention any difficulties you have experienced since living there – such as relationship or fertility problems. The practitioner assesses the surrounding environment to see if there are negative influences, such as a large tree casting a shadow on your home. Each room is assessed to determine if it has a positive or negative influence on your life. Some advice may seem strange: for example, it is considered bad luck to place your bed so your feet face the doorway. Other tips may feel like common sense: such as recommending that your home should be clutter-free.

# T'ai chi
The gentleness of t'ai chi exercise makes it ideal in pregnancy. It is a stylized form of martial art, performed in a controlled way so that you look as if you are dancing in slow motion.

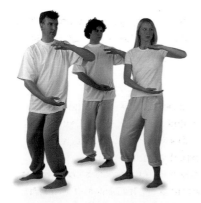

*T'ai chi trains the mind as well as the body. You have to focus on your posture in order to keep your movements smooth and co-ordinated.*

T'ai chi is based on the idea that our well-being depends on the circulation of energy through invisible channels (meridians) in the body – the same theory that is behind acupuncture. The smooth movements combine with breathing techniques to enhance this energy flow.

## SUITABLE FOR EVERYONE
T'ai chi can be done by anyone. It improves strength, posture and balance and also helps to keep joints flexible. Researchers have found that it can lower blood pressure and improve breathing technique – the latter being vital for labour. It may also help with backache, digestive problems and constipation. Once learned, it is very relaxing, and can be an effective method of relieving stress. T'ai chi is ideal for pregnant women because it is a gentle type of exercise with a calming influence, and its ability to develop physical and mental control can be of immense benefit when it comes to labour and birth.

There are several forms of t'ai chi. The type most commonly taught in the West is Yang style, short form. This consists of 24 linked movements, which take about five minutes to perform. Learning the movements properly takes time – you may spend a whole class on only one or two.

# Yoga

Many doctors and midwives now recommend yoga to pregnant women. It is known to foster general good health and improve posture and flexibility. It can also help to prevent or relieve backache, constipation and headaches.

Yoga is proven to help people relax, which makes it highly beneficial for pregnant women. Relaxation helps to improve the flow of blood, and so increases the supply of oxygen and nutrients to the baby. Yoga relaxation and breathing techniques can be very helpful during labour. Regular practice can help to strengthen the body, loosen up the pelvis in preparation for birth, and aid recovery afterwards.

Yoga has been practised for thousands of years in India and is now widely taught in the West. Most yoga practised by Westerners is a form of hatha yoga. This means that it involves physical postures (asanas) as well as breath-control techniques, meditation and relaxation exercises. Certain yoga poses, such as the spinal twists and headstands, should be avoided in pregnancy, so it is best to attend a class aimed specifically at pregnant women. Antenatal yoga classes are available in many areas for women in their second and third trimesters.

If you are pregnant and want to take up yoga for the first time, it is best to wait until you are past the 12-week mark before starting classes. If you already practise a regular, well-established yoga routine, it should be safe to continue in the first trimester, if you work gently and avoid unsuitable postures. Tell your teacher that you are pregnant.

## YOUR YOGA PRACTICE

In yoga, everyone works to his or her own capacity. Some people get into advanced postures easily; others are stiff and need to work with simplified versions. Do not push yourself further than you are naturally able to go. With practice, your body will become stronger and more flexible. In many classes, specialist equipment is available to help you with the postures. Yoga classes vary widely. Generally, they start with easy postures to warm up the body, then move on to more advanced ones. Usually, sitting, standing, reclining and some inversions (adapted if you are pregnant) are covered.

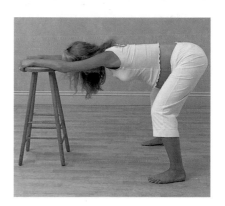

*Many yoga asanas need to be adapted for pregnancy. This woman is doing modified dog pose; the standard position would place a strain on her uterus.*

# Pilates

This form of body conditioning also develops mental awareness and an effective breathing technique. Pilates has parallels with yoga and, like yoga, can help alleviate back pain and other problems common in pregnancy.

Pilates aims to bring the body back to its natural alignment. The exercises encourage you to work to your maximum capability, without placing undue strain on the body. As a result, regular practice helps to improve your posture and flexibility, as well as toning the muscles. Pilates is particularly good for developing 'core' strength in the lower back and abdomen. It works the mind as well as the body, and many people find it deeply relaxing. Teachers say that almost anyone can practise Pilates because the exercises involved can be adapted to suit the individual's needs.

Pilates is safe for pregnant women as it uses carefully controlled movements and encourages you to work within your body's limitations. Advocates say that it can help to reduce backache, ease delivery and hasten recovery after the birth. However, it is important that the exercises are done correctly, so seek out a specialist qualified teacher who regularly works with pregnant women.

Pilates teachers say that it is important to practise three or four times a week in order to obtain the most benefit from this therapy.

## SAFE PILATES

- If you are pregnant and new to Pilates, do not start classes until after the first trimester. Try to find special pregnancy classes. Otherwise, go for individual instruction with an experienced teacher.
- Do not push your body any further than is comfortable: with practice, you will build up flexibility and strength.
- If you feel uncomfortable at any point, then always stop and rest.
- Do not do any exercises that require you to lie flat on your back after 30 weeks.
- Build up slowly – it will take time for you to increase your flexibility and strength.

# Alexander technique
This gentle posture-improver can lessen pressure on muscles and joints and ease many mental and physical problems.

As children, we have naturally good posture. However, as we grow up we tend to let bad habits become ingrained: we may slouch or cross our legs when we sit, for example. Our mental state, too, can affect our posture: when stressed we may hold our shoulders in a state of tension. Over time, poor posture causes damage to muscles and joints, and our digestive, respiratory and circulatory systems may also suffer.

## HOW IT HELPS
The Alexander technique trains people to stand and move in a better way. It emphasizes aligning the head with the spine, so that the neck remains free of strain. The technique is best taught on a one-to-one basis, with the teacher showing you how to perform a whole range of everyday tasks – such as getting in and out of a chair – in the Alexander way. The technique is accepted as an effective way of treating many back and neck problems, and is said to help people resist stress. Other conditions that may be eased include anxiety, depression, headaches, high blood pressure, infertility, breathing problems, fatigue, arthritis and digestive disorders.

The technique can help pregnant women cope with the back strain caused by carrying a 'bump' and will help you prepare for the birth. Alexander technique teaches women to stay upright during labour – in a squatting position – so that the force of gravity can assist the baby's passage. A practitioner will help you to learn how to cope with contractions without tensing the body. This can make childbirth easier, since tension increases pain.

# Osteopathy
Osteopaths believe that good health depends on the proper functioning of our muscles and joints.

Osteopaths work to correct imbalances caused by injury, poor posture and stress. Curative techniques include massage, limb stretches and sharp thrusts. You may hear a clicking sound as a joint slips back into alignment, but you should not feel any pain. Most people see an osteopath because of backache, but the therapy can also help with problems such as headaches, digestive disorders (common in pregnancy) and breathing difficulties. Osteopathy is safe in pregnancy, but only if performed by a qualified practitioner with experience in treating pregnant women.

Pregnant women are often advised to have regular sessions to help them adjust to changes in their posture as the baby grows, to prevent and treat lower back pain. Some osteopaths say that regular treatment during pregnancy can help to make the birth easier.

## CRANIAL OSTEOPATHY
Used to help many of the same conditions as conventional osteopathy, this uses delicate manipulation of the skull bones to improve blood and fluid circulation in the head.

# Chiropractic
Chiropractors believe that a well-aligned spine is vital for good health as it supports the body and houses the central nervous system.

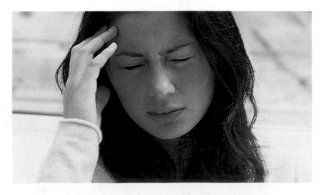

*Regular headaches may be relieved by releasing built-up tension in the spine through chiropractic.*

Chiropractic is mainly used to help with back and neck problems. Gentle manipulation of the spine is performed to improve posture, and to correct any kinks caused by injury or stress. Regular sessions of chiropractic can help pregnant women to adjust their posture so that they cope better with the strain of carrying a growing baby. It may also alleviate pelvic problems and make childbirth easier.

Chiropractics say that working on the spine can also help seemingly unrelated problems. This is because nerve pathways branch off the spine at different levels and travel to all areas of the body. Distortions in the spine can affect nerve function, and may therefore be the cause of problems elsewhere, such as fatigue, indigestion and constipation.

# Which therapy?

| | Here is a guide to which therapies may help certain conditions. You may need to experiment to find what works best for you. Always also get a diagnosis and any necessary treatment from your family doctor. | Herbalism p148 | Homeopathy p148 | Aromatherapy p149 | Massage p149 | Acupuncture p150 | Shiatsu p150 | Reflexology p150 | Meditation p151 | Hypnotherapy p151 | Reiki p151 | T'ai chi p152 | Yoga p153 | Pilates p153 | Alexander technique p154 | Osteopathy p154 | Chiropractic p154 |
|---|---|---|---|---|---|---|---|---|---|---|---|---|---|---|---|---|---|
| **Anxiety/Stress** | | • | • | • | • | • | • | | • | • | • | • | • | | | | |
| **Backache** | | | | • | • | • | • | • | | • | • | • | • | • | • | • | • |
| **Breastfeeding problems** | | • | • | | • | | | | | • | | | | | | | |
| **Breathlessness** | | | | | • | | | | | | • | • | • | • | • | • | |
| **Constipation** | | • | • | • | • | • | • | • | | | | • | • | | | • | • |
| **Cramps** | | • | • | • | • | | • | | | | | • | • | | | | |
| **Cystitis** | | • | • | | | • | • | | | | | | | | | | |
| **Dizziness** | | • | • | | • | • | • | | | | | • | • | • | | • | • |
| **Fatigue** | | • | • | • | • | • | • | • | • | • | • | • | • | • | | | |
| **Flatulence** | | • | • | • | • | | • | | | | | • | | | | | |
| **Haemorrhoids** | | • | • | • | • | • | • | • | | | | | | | | • | • |
| **Heartburn** | | • | • | | • | | | • | | | • | | | | | • | • |
| **Incontinence, urinary** | | • | • | | • | | | | | | | • | | | | | |
| **Insomnia** | | • | • | • | • | • | • | | • | • | • | • | • | | | | |
| **Labour** | | • | • | • | • | • | | • | | • | | • | | | | | |
| **Milk, insufficient supply of** | | • | • | | • | | | | | | | | | | | | |
| **Morning sickness** | | • | • | | | • | • | | • | • | • | • | | | | | |
| **Oedema** | | • | • | • | • | • | • | | | | | • | | | | | |
| **Pelvic discomfort** | | | | | • | • | | | | | | • | • | • | • | • | |
| **Perineal discomfort (postnatal)** | | • | • | • | | | | | | | | | | | | | |
| **Postnatal depression** | | • | • | • | • | • | | • | | | | • | | | | | |
| **Stretchmarks** | | • | • | • | • | | | | | | | | | | | | |
| **Sweating** | | • | • | | • | | | | | | | • | | | | | |
| **Thrush** | | • | • | • | | | • | | | | | | | | | | |
| **Urination (frequent)** | | • | • | | | | | | | | | • | | | | | |
| **Varicose veins** | | • | • | • | | • | | | | | | • | | | | | |

# Glossary

**Amniocentesis** This is a specialized test that involves taking fluid from the amniotic cavity (amnion). The amnion is the inner sac that surrounds the baby in the uterus. The cells contained within the fluid can be analysed and also grown in a tissue culture. Together the results provide information about chromosomal defects, the sex of the baby, inherited disorders, and open neural tube defects. *See pages 69–71.*

**Amniotic fluid** The fluid contained within the amnion. *See* **Amniocentesis**.

**Antenatal** This means before birth.

**Baby blues** *see* **postnatal depression**.

**Birth plan** With the help and co-operation of the hospital antenatal unit, you will be invited to draw up a birth plan, which states all of your wishes for the management of your labour and delivery.

**Braxton Hicks contractions** Painless contractions of the uterus that occur throughout pregnancy and more noticeably during the last trimester of pregnancy, when they may be mistaken for the contractions that signify impending birth.

**Breaking of the waters** The membranes surrounding the baby in the uterus rupture painlessly at the onset of labour, producing a gush of 'water'. The waters refer to the liquid contained within the membranes that surround the baby. Once the waters have broken, hospital admission or bed rest is advisable, since the baby is now no longer protected from infection or from any impact.

**Caesarean** A Caesarean section is performed by making an incision along the bikini line and lifting out the baby. This surgery is performed either with general anaesthetic or with an epidural. An **emergency** Caesarean is performed when it becomes clear that the baby cannot be born naturally and the need becomes urgent to deliver the baby quickly. An **elective** Caesarean is one in which the need for a Caesarean has been decided in advance.

**Chorionic villus sampling** This is a non-routine test carried out to detect fetal abnormality, and it is usually carried out at 9–10 weeks. A narrow tube is passed into the uterus, either through the vagina or through the abdomen, to the outer sac surrounding the baby, known as the chorion. A sample of the floating tendrils of the chorion, the villi, is sucked into the tube and analysed for information about the baby's genes. Ultrasound is used throughout the procedure to locate precisely the chorion and the villi. The test carries a risk of miscarriage.

**Colostrum** A milky fluid high in protein, minerals, vitamins and nitrogen, which precedes the flow of breast milk for two or three days after delivery. Colostrum also contains antibodies that bolster the baby's immune system, helping to fight infection.

**Dilation** The cervix gradually opens (dilates) to allow the baby's head to pass into the birth canal, and into the world.

**Eclampsia** *see* **pre-eclampsia**.

**Ectopic pregnancy** The fertilized egg implants not in the uterus but elsewhere in the abdomen or Fallopian tubes. Symptoms include bleeding and abdominal pain, sometimes severe, and pain in the shoulder. Immediate hospital admission is required.

**Embryo** The fertilized egg that eventually becomes the developing baby is known as the embryo for the first eight weeks of life. After that it is known as a fetus, until birth.

**Endorphins** The feel-good hormones that are released during exercise (and lovemaking) and continue to make us feel good and relieve pain for some time after the exercise itself has stopped.

**Engagement** The engagement of the baby's head in the upper part of the woman's pelvis. This usually occurs after the 36th week. (The pressure exerted by the baby's head is one of the factors that makes women need to urinate frequently in pregnancy.)

**Epidural** Local anaesthetic is injected into the epidural space between the spinal cord and the backbone of the lumbar region to provide total pain relief during labour and/or during a Caesarean. The baby is less likely to be affected by an epidural than by pethidine or general anaesthetic.

**Episiotomy** A surgical incision is made into the perineum (between the vagina and the anus) towards the end of the second stage of labour before the baby is born. The cut is made to relieve pressure on the muscle of the perineum, to prevent tearing of the muscle, to help the baby out, and if a forceps or ventouse delivery needs to be done.

**Fetoscopy** This procedure involves a microscope camera being inserted into the uterus through the abdomen in much the same way as amniocentesis so that the fetus can be photographed. By sampling tissue it may be possible to diagnose several blood and skin diseases that the amniocentesis test cannot. In some centres, certain fetal conditions can be treated before delivery by means of a fetoscopy. *See page 69.*

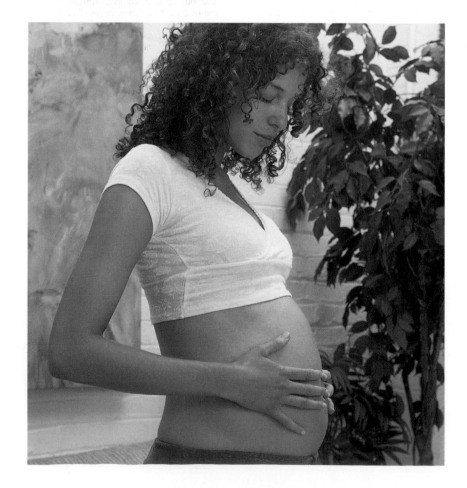

**Fetus** *see* **embryo**.

**Forceps** A pair of forceps looks like a pair of tongs or a pair of spoons. If there is a delay in the second stage of labour, they are passed up through the vagina and gently applied either side of the baby's head so that the baby can be drawn gently and slowly down the birth canal and delivered quickly. They are used when it can been seen that the baby needs some assistance, but that a Caesarean can still be avoided.

**Gas and air** Method of pain relief used during labour. The woman breathes in nitrous oxide and oxygen through a mouthpiece.

**Genetic counselling** Genetics is the science of heredity. Genetic counselling is offered to those couples who fail to conceive, who have repeated miscarriages or who have genetic disorders in their family medical histories.

**Induction** Labour can be induced artificially in hospital if it has become apparent that the baby needs to be born without delay but there is no sign of labour contractions starting. The three possible methods of induction include rupturing the membranes, administering pessaries and the use of a drip.

**Meconium** The faeces within the baby's rectum, meconium is composed of cellular debris, vernix and some lanugo, and is greenish-black in colour. If it is passed while the fetus is still in the uterus and under stress, it may discolour the amniotic fluid. The fluid's colour is carefully observed, therefore, when the waters break in order to detect any sign of meconium stain. If there is, this can signify fetal distress, necessitating the delivery of the baby without delay.

**Miscarriage** This is the lay (non-medical) term for the spontaneous loss of a pregnancy. A large percentage of pregnancies are lost, often for no known reason, sometimes before the woman even knows that she is pregnant. The medical term for miscarriage is spontaneous abortion.

**Morning sickness** Nausea and vomiting during pregnancy, commonly in the first trimester and commonly in the mornings, can occur throughout pregnancy and at any time of day. They are caused by hormonal changes, disturbing the normal metabolism of the body, by vascular changes leading to large variations in blood pressure; by upset to the digestive system caused by changes in the rates of secretion in the stomach and small intestine; and by psychological changes, which can produce anxiety.

**Neonatal** The period of four weeks immediately after the baby's delivery. A neonate is a newborn baby up to the age of four weeks.

**Nuchal fold ultrasound** The nuchal fold ultrasound is also sometimes known as the nuchal fold, the nuchal translucency test or the translucency scan. This is carried out at 11 to 14 weeks and is used to detect Down's syndrome cases. The procedure is as for a routine ultrasound, but the operator concentrates on getting a good image of the fetus's neck on the screen and measures a layer of fluid at the back of the neck. The thicker this layer is, the greater the chance the

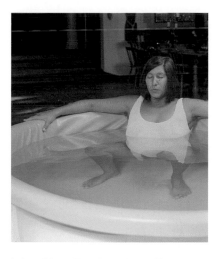

baby will have Down's syndrome. The chance or risk is expressed as a probability such as a one in 10,000 chance or a one in 100 chance.

**Oestrogen** This describes a number of hormones produced by the ovaries and the adrenal gland. During pregnancy, the placenta also produces oestrogen. The oestrogen hormones are responsible for the development of the female breasts and genitals at puberty and they also play a part in controlling the menstrual cycle. In pregnancy the hormones stimulate the growth of the uterus and breast tissue. *See also* **reproductive hormones**.

**Pethidine** A method of pain relief used in labour, this is an anaesthetic given by injection which lasts for three to four hours. It gives better pain relief than gas and air but is not as effective as an epidural.

**Placenta** The placenta is located within the uterus and to it is attached the fetus through the umbilical cord. The placenta provides the fetus with nutrients from the mother, eliminates fetal waste products and enables the fetus to breathe.

**Postnatal depression** Baby blues are common in new mothers. They may occur within five days of the birth and most women quickly recover from this temporary hormonal slump. Postnatal depression usually occurs later, even months after the birth. The mother's misery, fear and anger may be directed at herself, her baby or both. Irritability, fatigue and sleeplessness are characteristic. Professional help is needed. *See also pages 140–1.*

**Pre-eclampsia** This is the precursor to the very serious condition of convulsions in pregnancy, known as eclampsia. It is characterized by the development of high blood pressure, swelling (especially of the face, ankles and wrists), and by the appearance of protein in the urine. Urgent referral to hospital is required.

**Progesterone** One of the female hormones, progesterone is produced by the corpus luteum in the ovary, to a lesser extent by the adrenal gland, and in pregnancy by the placenta. It is responsible for building up the endometrium in the uterus, which feeds the developing embryo in the early days of pregnancy. Progesterone stimulates the

growth of the glandular, milk-producing tissue and helps smooth muscle to relax. *See also* **reproductive hormones**.

**Pudendal nerve block** Type of local anaesthetic injection that is used in labour. This method is used to numb the perineum, vagina and vulva prior to short, second stage labour procedures, such as forceps delivery and ventouse.

**Reproductive hormones** The menstrual cycle is controlled by the reproductive hormones, FSH (follicle-stimulating hormone) and LH (luteinizing hormone), which are released by the brain and which stimulate the ovaries to produce the female sex hormones, oestrogen and progesterone.

**Show** The first thing to happen at the beginning of labour is the appearance of a mucus plug from the vagina. This is known as a show of mucus and it is sometimes tinged with blood, which gives it a pinkish appearance. This is followed by the breaking of the waters, when hospital admission or bed rest are advised.

**Stillbirth** The death at or before the birth of the baby after 24 weeks' gestation. The term perinatal death, which doctors often use, includes stillbirth and the death of a baby in the first week of life.

**TENS** Transcutaneous Electrical Nerve Stimulation is a form of pain relief used during labour in which electrode pads discharging an electrical stimulus are placed on the woman's back. The woman controls the amount of electrical input with a hand-held control. Some women find it effective, while others do not. (TENS can also be used to relieve pain associated with many other medical conditions.)

**Termination** This is the medical or surgical ending of a pregnancy, which may be done for medical or social reasons. It is commonly known as abortion.

**Triple alphafetoprotein (AFP) test** Simple, safe and reliable blood test, taken between weeks 15 and 18, that yields information about the baby's health and development. *See pages 35, 68–9.*

**Ultrasound** This enables the fetus to be viewed in the uterus, providing useful information about the baby's health and development at different stages from week seven of gestation.

**Umbilical cord** This connects the fetus to the placenta, from which it derives nourishment. After the baby has been delivered, the cord is clamped and cut. The umbilical stump remains, protruding from the baby's navel, then shrivels and eventually falls off towards the end of the first week of life.

**Ventouse suction** Also known as vacuum extraction, this is a last-minute medical assistance with delivery, which is carried out when the baby is in difficulties. A small cup is passed up the vagina and attached by suction to the baby's head, suction being induced by means of a small hand pump. The cup is then gently pulled to help the baby down the birth canal.

# Useful addresses and websites

## UNITED KINGDOM

**Miscarriage Association**
Clayton Hospital
Northgate, Wakefield
West Yorkshire WF1 3JS
tel: 01924 200799
www.the-ma.org.uk

**The Multiple Births Foundation**
Queen Charlotte's and Chelsea
Hospital
Du Cane Road
London W12 0HS
tel: 020 8383 3519
www.multiplebirths.org.uk

**National Childbirth Trust**
Alexander House
Oldham Terrace
Acton
London W3 6NH
tel: 0870 4448707
breastfeeding support line:
0870 4448707
www.nctpregnancyandbabycare.com

**Relate** (relationship counselling)
Herbert Gray College
Little Church Street
Rugby
Warwickshire CV21 3AP
tel: 01788 573241
Helpline: 0845 1304010
www.relate.org.uk

**Royal College of Obstetricians
and Gynaecologists**
27 Sussex Place
London NW1
tel: 020 7772 6200
www.rcog.org.uk

**The British Register of
Complementary Practitioners
(BRCP)**
Institute for Complementary
Medicine
PO Box 194
London SE16 7QZ
tel: 020 7237 5165
www.icmedicine.co.uk

## UNITED STATES

**The American College of
Obstetricians and Gynecologists**
409 12th Street NW
Washington DC
200024-2188
tel: 202 638 5577
www.acog.org

**National Association of
Childbearing Centers**
3123 Gottschall Road
Perkiomenville PA 18074
tel: 215 234 8068
www.birthcenters.org

**National Women's Health Network**
514 10th Street NW
Washington DC 20004
tel: 202 347 1140
www.womenshealthnetwork.org

**American Holistic Medical
Association**
12101 Menaul Blvd., NE, Suite C
Albuquerque
NM 87112
tel: 505 292 7788
www.holisticmedicine.org

## CANADA

**Canadian Examining Board of
Health** Care Practitioners Inc
658 Danforth Avenue
Suite 204, Toronto

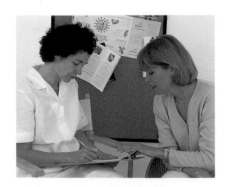

Ontario M4J 5B9
www.canadianexaminingboard.com

**Canadian Women's Health
Network**
Suite 203, 419 Graham Avenue
Winnipeg, Manitoba R3C 0M3
tel: 204 942 5500
www.cwhn.ca

## AUSTRALIA

**Australian Complementary
Health Association**
247 Flinders Lane
Melbourne, Vic 3000
tel: (03) 9650 5327
fax: (03) 9650 8404
www.diversity.org.au

**Australian Women's Health
Network**
www.awhn.org.au

## NEW ZEALAND

**The New Zealand Health
Information Network**
PO Box 337
Christchurch 8015
tel: 03 980 4646
www.nzhealth.net.nz

## SOUTH AFRICA

www.childbirth.co.za
www.activebirth.co.za

**African Health Anthology**
www.nisc.co.za

## INTERNATIONAL
WEBSITES

www.pregnancy.com
www.activebirthcentre.com
www.homebirth.org.uk
www.mothers35plus.co.uk

# Index

acupuncture, 16, 40, 41, 73, 74, 75, 83, 99, 111, 119, 127, 141, 150
ailments, 40–1, 60–1, 74–5, 98–9
air travel, 25
alcohol, 24, 95
Alexander technique, 45, 74, 75, 79, 99, 154
alphafetoprotein test, 36, 68–9
amenorrhoea, 10
amniocentesis, 36, 69, 70–1, 72, 73, 77
antenatal care, 34–5
    checks, 66–7, 76, 94–5
    team, 35
    tests, 35, 36–7, 42, 68–9, 76
antenatal classes, 96–7
anxiety, 18, 40, 53, 61, 66, 84, 100, 127
    calming exercise, 127
Apgar score, 132
aromatherapy, 16, 54–5, 57, 74, 79, 83, 99, 111, 141, 146, 149
    first aid, 55
assisted delivery, 124–5

baby, 130–45
    common problems, 142–3
    danger symptoms, 143
    feeding, 134–5
    holding and handling, 133
    newborn, 123, 132–3
    sleeping, 141
baby blues, 140
baby clothes and equipment, 112–13
Bach Flower Remedies, 61, 111, 127
backache/pain, 29, 45, 50, 57, 62, 74, 79, 92, 99, 126
Bart's test, 69
bathing baby, 138
birth, 97, 100, 102–29
    medical interventions, 124–5

positions, 121–3
    preparing for, 110–11
    recovering from, 140
birth marks, 133
birth partner, 101, 105, 120, 129
birth plan, 104–5
birthing pool, 108–9, 119
bleeding, 11, 27, 40
blood tests, 67
body changes, 16–17, 50–1, 82–3
bonding, 19, 53, 101, 103, 133
bottle-feeding, 134, 136
    cleaning equipment, 137
breastfeeding, 134–6, 144
breasts, 16, 17, 40, 50
    massage, 89
breathing techniques in labour, 110–11
breathlessness, 82–3, 98, 99
breech baby, 114, 115, 126
burping baby, 136

Caesarean, 67, 114, 124–5, 128
calcium, 20, 21–2, 98
carbohydrates, 20
career see work
carsickness, baby's 145
cats, 24, 25, 145
cervix dilation, 117, 122
chemicals, 25
chiropractic, 50, 74, 75, 99, 154
chloasma, 51
chorionic villus sampling, 36, 68, 72
clothes, 50, 86
colds and flu, 55, 143
colic, 142
colour therapy, 151
confirming pregnancy, 10–11
constipation, 22, 74, 143, 
contractions, 101, 117, 128
    Braxton Hicks, 82, 83, 117
    induced birth, 128
cooking, 32–3
cordocentesis, 69
cot death, 141
coughs, 143
counselling, 73, 85
cradle cap, 142
cramp, 98
cranial osteopathy, 145
croup, 143
crying, 142
crystal healing, 151
cystitis, 67, 75

dance therapy, 26–7
delivery date, 10, 68
delivery room, 117
depression, 100
    postnatal, 140–1
diabetes, 66, 67, 94
diarrhoea, 143

diet, 16, 20–3, 41, 51, 74, 98, 99, 110
    foods to avoid, 24–5
dogs, 24, 145
Domino scheme, 34
Doppler ultrasound, 36
Down's syndrome, 36, 71
    tests, 36, 68, 69, 70
dried formula feeds, 137

eclampsia, 67, 94
ectopic pregnancy, 11, 38
embryo, 12–15
emotions, 18–19, 52–3, 60, 82, 84–5
    postnatal, 131, 140–1
    and termination, 73
engagement, 83
environmental hazards, 25
episiotomy, 124, 140
essential oils, 54–5, 111, 127
    see also aromatherapy
exercise, 16, 26–7, 86
expressing breast milk, 136
eye infections, 143

face massage, 59, 89
fainting, 40
family doctor, 8, 11, 17, 34, 35, 40, 41, 75, 99, 107
father/father-to-be see partner
fatigue, 16, 40, 44, 52, 140, 145
feeding baby, 134–5
feet, 51, 55
feng shui, 152
fetal abnormality, 71, 72
fetal blood sampling, 69
fetal monitoring, 119
fetoscopy, 69
fetus, 13, 14–15, 46–9, 66, 68, 80–1
fibre, 22
first trimester, 8–43
fish, 20, 24
folic acid, 22, 23
food cravings, 10, 17
foods, harmful, 24–5
forceps delivery, 124
fruit and vegetables, 20, 110
    juices, 9, 16

genetic counselling, 37
German measles see rubella
going public, 42, 47
Guthrie tests, 133

haemorrhoids, 75, 126, 140
hair, 51, 86
handling new baby, 133
head exercises, 28
headaches, 28, 40, 55, 56, 75
herbal teas, 40, 41, 60, 99, 111, 135

teas to avoid, 60
herbalism, 41, 74, 75, 99, 142, 148
hereditary disorders, 37, 70
high blood pressure, 56, 66, 67, 94, 99
hip exercises, 29
home, 32, 33
    aromatherapy, 55
    massage, 57
home delivery, 34, 106–7, 109
    what you will need, 107
homeopathy, 41, 61, 74–5, 99, 111, 127, 148
    for baby, 142
    breastfeeding, 135
    turning breech baby, 126
hormones, 44, 51, 52, 140
hospital birth, 34, 106
    booking-in appointment, 34
    going to hospital, 117
    what to take, 106
human chorionic gonadotrophin, 10–11, 69
hypnotherapy, 151

incontinence, 17, 83, 98
indigestion, 60, 75, 99
induction, 124, 126, 128
insomnia, 40, 54, 56
iron, 20, 21, 110

joints, keeping mobile 28–9

kidney disease, 67, 94

labour, 102, 116
    assessment for, 114
    length of, 117
    pain relief, 118–19
    positions for, 119, 122–3
    preparing for, 101, 110–11
    stages of, 101, 117, 120–3
    start of, 116–17
late baby, 126–7
leg exercises, 29
leg massage, 58, 99
length of pregnancy, 78
lie, baby's, 114–15
lifestyle, 32–3, 86–7
linea nigra, 51
listeriosis, 24–5
livestock, 25

massage, 40, 56–7, 83, 119, 149
    abdomen, 89
    aromatherapy, 16, 54–5, 57
    back, 57, 74, 99
    breast, 89
    facial, 59, 89
    leg, 58, 99
    with partner, 41, 57, 86
    perineal, 88–9
    self-massage, 58–9, 86

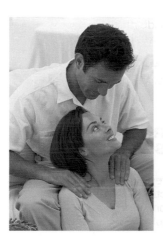

shoulder, 59, 75
  Swedish, 149
  when to avoid, 57
meat and poultry, 20, 24
meditation, 40, 99, 119, 127, 147, 151
midwife, 34, 35, 40, 84, 106, 117
migraines, 75
milk and dairy products, 20, 24
minerals, 20, 23
miscarriage, 38–9, 44, 52, 70, 71
  causes, 39
  early and late, 39
  warning signs, 38
monitoring in labour, 119
morning sickness see nausea
moxibustion, 126
multiple pregnancy, 15, 37

nappies, 138
  changing, 138–9
nappy rash, 138, 142
natural therapies, 60–1, 87, 111 146–55
  choosing, 155
nausea, 16–17, 41, 44, 50, 52
neck exercises, 28
nipples, 16, 51, 89, 144
nuchal fold ultrasound, 35, 36, 68
nutrition see diet

older mother, 37
  and amniocentesis, 70, 71
organic food, 21
osteopathy, 50, 74, 75, 99, 154

pain relief, 105, 110, 118–19, 128
partner, 16, 42, 52
  bonding, 19, 53, 101, 133
  going off sex, 64, 65
  involvement, 19, 53, 84–5, 96
  massage, 41, 57, 86
  presence at birth, 105, 109, 120, 129
  spending time with, 65, 84
pelvic floor exercises, 29, 98
perineal massage, 88–9
period, missed, 10

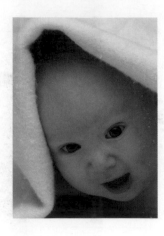

pigmentation, 51
Pilates, 27, 50, 74, 99, 110, 127, 153
placenta, 13, 22, 46
  delivery of, 123
position, baby's, 114–15
positions, birth 121–3
positive thinking, 87
postnatal depression, 140–1
posture, 29, 45, 79
  and backache, 50, 74, 99
  exercises, 30–1, 62
pre-eclampsia, 67, 94, 99
pregnancy test, 10–11
premature baby, 78, 95
presentation, baby's, 114–15
protein, 21, 110
pubic joint pain, 99

radiation, 25
reflexology, 75, 83, 87, 99 127, 150
reiki, 41, 74, 75, 79, 87, 99, 127, 151
risk factors, 37, 107
rubella, 70

salmonella, 25
salt, 24
scan see ultrasound scan

sciatica, 29, 62, 92
second trimester, 44–77
sex during pregnancy, 64–5, 77, 85
shiatsu, 87, 150
shoulders,
  exercises, 28
  massage, 59, 75
show, 101, 116, 117
silica, 51
single parent, 129
skin problems, 99
  baby's, 133
sleep, 16, 95, 98
  baby's patterns, 141
  lack of, 141
spina bifida, 22, 68, 70
spine, loosening up, 29
stress, 10, 95, 100
  de-stress, 28, 54, 127
stretching exercises, 28–9
  perineal stretch, 91
  in water, 26, 92–3
  yoga, 30–1, 62
stretchmarks, 41, 51, 55, 74, 89
sudden infant death syndrome, 141
sugar, 20, 24
supplements, 23
swimming, 16, 26, 41, 86
swollen ankles/feet/legs, 56, 67, 94, 98, 99

t'ai chi, 27, 99, 152
taste, 17
TENS, 118, 119
termination, 71, 72–3, 77
third trimester, 78–101
thrush, 75
tiredness see fatigue
touch, 56, 86, 101
toxic substances, avoidance of, 24–5
toxoplasmosis, 25, 69
transitional stage, 120
transverse lie, 114, 115, 126
twins, 15, 37, 43, 78, 101, 109, 123, 126

ultrasound scan, 11, 15, 37
  32-week, 95
  Doppler, 36
  first, 11, 15, 35
  mid-pregnancy, 49, 68
  nuchal fold, 35, 36, 68
umbilical cord, 13, 132
urinary infections, 41, 67, 75
urination, frequent, 16, 17, 41, 50, 83
urine tests, 11, 67
uterus, 16, 17, 29, 50, 83, 99, 117

vaginal discharge, 41
varicose veins, 26, 57, 74
ventouse extraction, 124
vernix, 48–9
visualization, 53, 110, 119, 120, 127
vitamins, 20, 22, 23, 51
vomiting, 17, 41, 143

walking, 16, 22, 26, 41, 51, 86, 126
water, 98, 110, 119
  exercising in, 26, 92–3
  retention, 99
water birth, 108–9, 119
waters breaking, 101, 116
weight,
  antenatal checks, 66
  gain, 23, 51
  overweight, 11, 66
work 33, 43, 110

X-rays, 25

yoga, 27, 45, 74, 96, 110, 153
  aqua yoga, 26, 92–3
  first trimester, 30–1
  second trimester, 50, 62–3
  third trimester, 79, 86, 90–3, 98, 99, 126, 127

zinc, 20, 22, 51

## ACKNOWLEDGEMENTS

**Anne Charlish:**
I am grateful to Mr Donald Gibb, to Professor Gedis Grudzinskas and Patricia Roberts for their assistance over many years on the subjects of pregnancy and birth.

**Publisher:**
The Publishers are grateful to the following picture libraries for permission to reproduce the photographs listed below in this book (all those not listed below are © Anness Publishing Ltd): t=top; b=bottom; c=centre; l=left; r=right

*Science Photo Library:*
p15 tr P. Saada/Eurelios; p34 b /Ruth Jenkinson/MIDIRS; p49 tl /Neil Bromhall; p67 tr /Faye Norman; p72 b /Hank Morgan; p95 bl /Ian Hooton; p96 b /Ruth Jenkinson/MIDIRS; p107 tl /Mark Clarke; p109 t /Petit Format; p119 tr /Ruth Jenkinson/MIDIRS; p124 /Tracy Dominey; p125 br /Hank Morgan; p126 tr /Mark de Fraeye; p132 /Simon Fraser; p133 bl /BSIP, Astier; p134 tr /BSIP, Astier

*Corbis:*
p37 t /Tom and Dee Ann McCarthy; p45 tr /Angela Wood; p45 br /Larry Williams and Associates; p81 tr /Larry Williams; p105 br /Douglas Kirkland; p123 br /Larry Williams; p130 Corbis only; p133 tr /Ariel Skelley; p141 /Susan Solie Patterson

The publishers would also like to thank:
MOT Models agency; Pregnant Pause Agency; the Warehouse studio (location setting); Bridget Baker for advice; Bonieventure Bagalue for assisting photographer Alistair Hughes; Sue Duckworth for helping with props; Born in Bristol for nappies and advice; Chris Bernstein for the index; Doriel Hall and Françoise Freedman for use of material, which we have adapted, on yoga and massage (mainly pp30/1, 62/3, 58/9, 90/1 and 92/3).

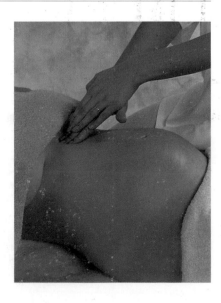